the Anti-Aging Fitness
PRESCRIPTION

the Anti-Aging Fitness
PRESCRIPTION

A day-by-day nutrition and workout plan to age-proof your body and mind

Z. Altug, MS, PT
Tracy Olgeaty Gensler, MS, RD

Foreword by Dennis McCullough, MD,
Dartmouth Medical School

Photos by Peter Field Peck

Healthy Living Books
New York • London

A Healthy Living Book
Hatherleigh Press
5-22 46th Avenue, Suite 200
Long Island City, NY 11101
www.healthylivingbooks.com

Library of Congress Cataloging-in-Publication data

Altug, Z.
 The anti-aging fitness prescription / Z. Altug, Tracy Olgeaty Gensler.
  p. cm.
 Includes bibliographical references.

ISBN-13: 978-1-57826-215
ISBN-10: 1-57826-215-1

 1. Exercise. 2. Aging--Physiological aspects. 3. Physical fitness. 4.
Longevity. I. Gensler, Tracy Olgeaty. II. Title.
 RA781.A48 2005
 362.17--dc22
        2005031502

All forms of exercise pose some inherent risks. The information in this book is meant to supplement, not replace, proper exercise training. Before practicing the exercises in this book, be sure that your equipment is well maintained. Do not take risks beyond your level of experience, training, and fitness. The exercise and dietary programs in this book are not intended as a substitute for any exercise routine or treatment or dietary regimen that may have been prescribed by your doctor. As with all exercise and dietary programs, you should get your doctor's approval before beginning. The author(s), editors, and publisher advise readers to take full responsibility for their safety and know their limits.

This publication contains the opinions and ideas of its authors only. The views and opinions of authors expressed herin do not necessarily state or reflect those of the University of California, and shall not be used for advertising or product endorsement purposes.

All Healthy Living Books are available for bulk purchase, special promotions, and premiums. For information about reselling and special purchase opportunities, please call 1-800-528-2550 and ask for the Special Sales Manager.

Cover design by Deborah Miller.
Interior design by Deborah Miller and Jacinta Monniere.

10 9 8 7 6 5 4 3 2 1

Printed in Canada

Contents

Foreword

At present, according to the U.S. Census Bureau, there are 50,000 centenarians in the United States. By the year 2050, demographers say, the number of Americans age 100 and older will soar to 800,000. In the meantime, the nation's 77 million Baby Boomers have begun retiring. Just what kind of shape will they be in? Geriatricians, doctors who treat senior citizens, are quaking in fearful anticipation of the coming deluge of elders. Why? Because so many have waited too long to take their physical health and diet seriously.

If you're afraid of becoming one of those overweight, unfit, homebound seniors, this book is for you. *The Anti-Aging Fitness Prescription* gives you a lively and proven practical program for engaging and improving your health in your 30s, 40s, 50s and far beyond. I'm a geriatrician who has been a physician for an elite group of seniors aged 65 to 105 at Kendal-at-Hanover, one of America's finest senior living communities, and I've seen your future. As one of my patients put it, sitting in my office in his still sweaty exercise clothes, "For the first half of your life, you can get away with neglect and even abuse your body; then, you'd better get serious about caring for yourself." At 83, Joe is lean, energetic, and bright-eyed and still moves with quickness in his step. Although he does have some arthritis, mild high blood pressure, and a "weathering" exterior, we both noted that he still doesn't need Viagra . . . or a lot of other medications his peers depend upon.

Joe is one of many older patients I have cared for who decided that later life could feel better than a downhill slide. Never athletic in his early years, committed to family and work responsibilities in adulthood, he nevertheless made a choice to try what we might now call a "makeover." And he succeeded. Now, he is no longer toiling in the middle of the pack, but way out in front of his peers, someone with the wisdom and determination to improve his well-being in later life.

Did it happen overnight? No, it was hard work at the start, but once he had the taste of better things and a set of habits that he came to associate with improved wellbeing (and the respect and envy of his friends), he rarely looked back. Can everyone do it so easily and successfully? Probably not.

However, you *can* do it, and *The Anti-Aging Fitness Prescription* is the perfect guide to your new lifestyle. The depth of information and the options for bringing real change to your health are all laid out here in an easy-to-follow eight-week program. Each day the program explores topics that will have you thinking and feeling differently (and more intelligently) about food. Similarly, exercises directed toward improved stamina, strength, flexibility, and balance will re-acquaint you with the potentials of your body and the increasing pleasure that comes with the discipline of regular use. Having worked with older folks who are "re-tooling" in our Senior Fitness Program at Dartmouth Medical School, I can literally guarantee you that making a hard run at this eight-week program will take you to a new, healthier place in your life. I will be using this program and recommending it to family, friends, and patients as a way of getting to another level of wellness.

Being an old athlete myself, I have always enjoyed reading in lay magazines about nutrition and exercise. What is new for me as a practicing and teaching physician of many years is that I can now pick up a medical journal and read still another study pointing up the proven value of better nutrition and exercise—*at all ages*! How do you deal with early joint pains and problems? Better diet and exercise! How do you counteract the tendency toward diabetes, high cholesterol levels, or elevated blood pressure? Better diet and exercise! How do elder patients live better lives, walking more steadily, sleeping better, experiencing less pain, being more engaged—even when they reside in a nursing home? Better diet and exercise! The evidence is in—this is no longer a matter of speculation.

From the moment you are born, you begin aging. No one can stop that. But you can control how you will feel and what you can do as you age. You do the math—where are you in your aging and where do you want to be? Perhaps it's time for a program that lets you know how it *feels* to be aging well. Become an inspiration, model, and resource for your friends—take this book and get started soon.

Dennis McCullough, MD
Associate Professor
Community Geriatric Consultant
Senior Fitness Program
Dartmouth Medical School
Hanover, NH

Acknowledgements

We would like to thank our patients who inspired us and made many great suggestions for this book.

Thanks to Kevin Moran, for believing in this project. Thanks to our wonderful editor, Andrea Au, for her patience, guidance, and attention to detail throughout the writing process, and the entire Hatherleigh team, including Andrew Flach, Deborah Miller, Alyssa Smith, and Erin Byram, for bringing this book to life. Thanks also to our photographer Peter Field Peck, model Andrea Sooch, and consultant James Villepigue.

Z would like to especially thank John Caramico, strength and conditioning coaches Al Miller and David Van Halanger, his professors at West Virginia University (Rachel A. Yeater and William L. Alsop) and the University of Pittsburgh (Sue Whitney), Janet Tucay, and Ellen Wilson at the UCLA Medical Center, and his brother Aykut Altug for their guidance and support.

We'd like to thank Nancy Clark, MS, RD, a sports nutritionist in Boston, for bringing us together as a writing team. Finally, a big thank you to our families for all their encouragement through the years.

ix

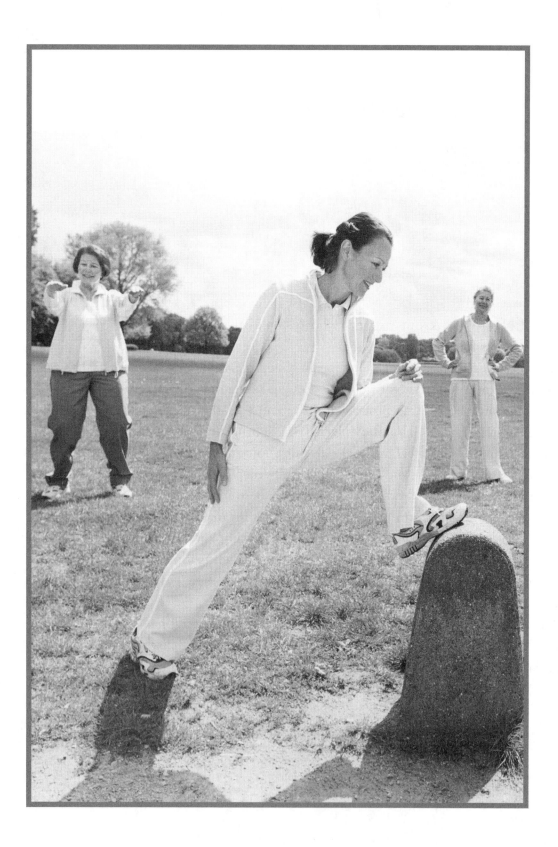

Introduction

Welcome to Your Anti-Aging Fitness Prescription

So what is the secret to maintaining a sharp mind and a fit, able body as you age? Much of what we thought were unavoidable symptoms of aging, such as loss of muscle mass, failing memory, balance problems, vision loss, and insomnia, can actually be avoided with the right plan. Physical fitness plays a major role in your health, improving your ability to move about with ease and perform daily tasks of living such as grocery shopping, cooking, mowing the lawn, gardening, and keeping your home in good repair. Good nutrition can help preserve your vision, maintain bone density, and manage diseases like hypertension, type 2 diabetes, and heart disease.

Maybe you associate wrinkles and gray hair with aging. Aging is a fact of life and it begins the minute you're born. We don't see too many babies with wrinkles, but aging begins just the same. We experience cellular and molecular adjustments as time moves on, very gradual changes that affect the structure and function of our brain, nerves, heart and blood vessels, immune response, bone and muscle, virtually every aspect of our body. The goal of this book is to help you ease these transitions, age successfully, and be able to enjoy each day that you are alive.

We all know someone who gradually moved more slowly as she got older. A broken bone after a fall or surgery left her weakened and dependent on a wheelchair or walker, and slowly, she lost her independence. She couldn't shop for groceries, go to the hairdresser, or keep doctors'

1

appointments without help from others to drive and guide her around. Every outing seemed to require so much planning that she stopped leaving the house entirely. She worried about her balance and feared falling and injuring herself. As a result, she began to move around the house less and less. You vow never to let that happen to you. But what are you doing to prevent it?

The loss of strength can happen earlier than you expect. Have you ever been unusually sore after a day of gardening or cleaning the house? This is one sign that you need to get moving. We witnessed a 50ish woman at the appliance store deciding on which cook-top to buy. She refused to purchase one model because the burner grates were too heavy for her to move. They only weighed about five pounds each, but to her they might as well have been 50 pounds because she couldn't budge them. When you lose the ability to perform simple tasks that used to be easy for you, improving your physical fitness should become a top priority.

Facts often flood the media with conflicting advice about exercise. Should I be walking or running, indoors or out, and should I be shooting for my fat-burning or cardio heart rate? Thirty minutes of exercise a day or is it 60, and what type of exercise are they expecting us to do? The message doesn't need to be so muddled. As health professionals, we sympathize with your confusion over these mixed messages. We'll set the record straight on what exercises will keep you healthy as you age. You'll have guidelines on the types of exercise and the

intensity and duration that you should do to improve your range of motion (reach for that can on the top shelf), flexibility (bend over and pick up the car keys you dropped), and strength (carry groceries). Through our day-to-day activity map, you'll be armed with all of the information you need to follow our simple steps for success.

Dieting is a multi-billion-dollar industry. Fad diets are increasingly popular, and we tend to focus more on trying to lose weight than on making changes that contribute to our health and fit into our lifestyle. And maintaining weight loss doesn't seem to be a priority as long as the weight comes off easily. Whether you have weight to lose or not, eating more fruits and vegetables is going to help you stay healthy inside and out. It's hard to gain weight with at least six servings a day of colorful produce, and the health benefits of consuming fruits and vegetables every day are endless. They contribute water to your intake, which is essential for the many chemical reactions in your body; the soluble fiber lowers blood cholesterol levels and helps you feel full with fewer calories; and the phytochemicals can fight a variety of diseases. Your three servings of calcium-rich foods will ramp up your calcium intake to help maintain bone health and manage hypertension. The nutrition diaries in Part II will map out easy, healthy meals and snacks incorporating these recommendations.

Our Anti-Aging Formula

There are many so-called remedies for anti-aging, such as supplements and herbs, that can be expensive and dangerous. If it sounds too good to be true, it probably is. We've all seen the commercials for specialized exercise machines that promise a 20-year-old's physique. Some scientific studies even recommend drastic measures such as walking around half-starved on too few calories in order to live a few years longer. We don't think you want to drastically limit your calories to the brink of starvation and forego the enjoyment of eating forever only to get a little more mileage out of your body. Holidays, family gatherings, and parties offer food traditions that we look forward to all year long. Food is a part of every get-together, and it's critical to maintain your energy for exercise. It would be foolish to suggest that you overhaul your lifestyle for anti-aging. The steps we recommend are simple, achievable options that are easy to maintain and will improve your quality of life a*t any age.*

Our approach promises that you won't have to take special potions, lotions, and pills and you won't have to exercise using expensive gadgets and gizmos. The theme throughout our book is that feeling good and being healthy is not a random event. A little effort and planning go a long way. Our anti-aging formula focuses on eating wholesome foods, getting sensible exercise, sleeping enough, controlling your stress, including laughter into your day, getting plenty of fresh air and a little sunshine, having healthy relationships with your family and friends, having a job that you enjoy, and, finally, maintaining a positive attitude. As for

nutritional supplements, we only advocate them in certain circumstances (such as a medically documented dietary deficiency and, for some people, we recommend vitamin D supplementation). Ideally, they should be used under the guidance of your physician and dietitian for safety and effectiveness, especially if you are taking medications or have a medical condition.

So here's the program in a nutshell:

Exercise regularly. Use our Perfect Triangle Prescription. Find at-home strength, flexibility, and aerobic exercises you can stick with.

Shoot for three. Have at least three meals a day, three calcium-rich foods, and three different colored vegetables and fruits every day to get your phytochemicals and critical nutrients for anti-aging.

Manage your stress. Identify and eliminate stressors from your life and try diaphragmatic breathing or yoga techniques to control daily stress.

Get enough sleep. Drowsy people perform poorly at school and work and cause car accidents. Recent research shows that sleep debts can cause impaired carbohydrate metabolism, possibly linked to type 2 diabetes. Achieve a restful night's sleep with proper sleep positioning and an appropriate pillow and mattress. Identify ways to make more sleep a priority, relax at bedtime, and fall asleep easier.

Get enough vitamin D. Choose vitamin D-rich foods or plan some time in the sun to synthesize vitamin D. Adequate vitamin D can be beneficial for prevention of breast, colon, and prostate cancer, some autoimmune diseases such as multiple sclerosis, and improvement in mood and symptoms of depression and more restful sleep.

Your approach towards making these changes should be gradual. A lifetime of stress-inducing habits isn't going to be erased in a day. A good night's sleep may require some changes that take time and patience. And we all know how hard it can be to clear out your cabinets for the latest "diet," reclassifying foods as good or bad, right or wrong. We don't even attempt this. The food recommendations are simple and sensible. You'll find a variety of exercises that will give you options you hadn't even considered before. The activity maps and nutrition diaries in Part II provide you with a structure that spells out your plan step by step. All of our advice is backed by scientific studies in peer-reviewed journals, and many of the findings have stood the test of time. You can embrace this healthy, sensible lifestyle gradually by using the steps outlined in the activity maps and nutrition diaries. Follow the Eight-Week Anti-Aging Fitness Prescription in Part II to guide you slowly but surely towards the most important lifestyle changes for anti-aging.

While we can't keep you from looking for the early bird special or retiring to Florida—and of course we can't really turn back or stop time, we *can* give you a solid foundation to preserve your health along the way and counteract the effects of aging.

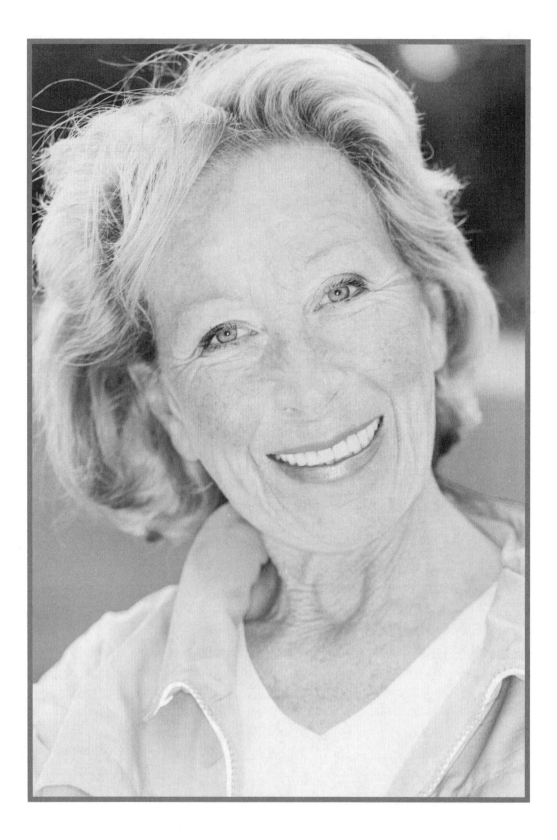

Part I

The Elements of Your Anti-Aging Prescription

You wake up too early to the sound of the neighbor's dog barking incessantly. You grumble, turn over, and try to go back to sleep, but it's no use; you're up for the day now. You stumble into the shower, agonize about the full day ahead of you, nine hours of work, a church meeting at night, and planning your sister's surprise birthday party after that. This schedule doesn't leave much time for sleep and de-stressing.

These are important factors for fighting the negative aspects of aging. As we see it, anti-aging is about enjoying lifelong good health, having the energy and ability to perform daily tasks of living, and making time for what's really important. It's never too late to start implementing our recommendations to realize greater enjoyment in your life.

Sleep is essential to refresh from a full day's worth of activity, particularly muscle repair and rejuvenation after exercise. Athletic performance studies find that sleep debts lead to a reduction in athletic performance, reaction time, and the ability to process information. Also, workouts seem harder and your anger threshold is lowered, leaving you snapping at people and easily dissatisfied.

Our technologically advanced lifestyle of 24-hour shopping, internet surfing, cable television and yapping on our cell phone has added stress to our life. Stress is connected to hypertension, inflammation, and a host of diseases. Exercise reduces stress and improves mood as well as quality of life. Our relaxation techniques including diaphragmatic breathing or positive mental imagery are helpful for de-stressing.

Your time is your own. It is possible to prioritize your day to make some changes that allow you enough shut-eye and leave a little breathing room in your schedule for calm, stress-free time. Part I describes the health benefits of managing stress and catching Z's, as well as the exercises and recipes you'll need to put your plan in place. The activity maps and nutrition diaries in Part II will give you day-by-day guidance to gradually introduce these principles into your lifestyle.

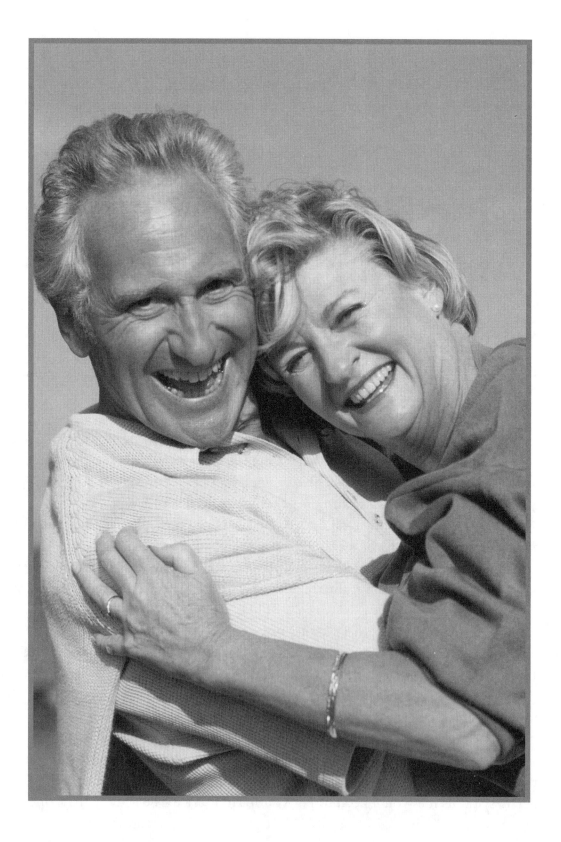

Chapter 1

Your Anti-Aging Lifestyle Guide

What is the Aging Process?

As we age, we experience changes in how we look and feel. There is a general decline in cellular activity and organ systems slow down. This can mean wrinkles and hair loss as well as disease. Everyone handles these changes differently, and they don't necessarily have to result in an aging appearance or a slower pace of life. Exercise can offset some of these changes by improving blood flow, preserving and building muscle mass, and improving digestion, respiratory, and skeletal health.

Regular physical activity can decelerate the aging process and improve antibody response in adults over 65. Aerobic activity may reduce brain tissue loss which is a normal part of aging. Strength, balance, and agility training (such as the Very Slow Motion Balancing and Walking in Place on page 82, Dancer's Balance on page 83, Heel Raises on page 62, or the March in Place on page 31) improve your reflexes, and your postural control, so that you are less likely to fall.

Neurodegenerative diseases, often associated with aging, are marked by a loss of memory, mobility, independence, or wellbeing. Neurodegeneration is the loss of spinal cord neurons and brain neurons (or cells). These cells help you make decisions, control movement and process sensory information. Neuron damage or loss can have overwhelming effects on your body as it ages, including Alzheimer's, Parkinson's or Huntington's disease, multiple sclerosis and amyotrophic lateral sclerosis (ALS). Exercise is a protective factor against neurodegeneration.

In 2003, the Department of Health and Human Services Administration on Aging recommended that all Americans increase their physical activity as an essential part of aging with vigor. The National Center for Chronic Disease Prevention and Health Promotion advocates regular physical activity, healthy eating, and avoidance of tobacco as the best-known prevention measures for healthy aging. So what are we waiting for? Let's get started!

Improve Your Sleep

Sleep is probably the most underrated aspect of maintaining good health. Many folks have long-term sleep deprivation, which can lead to a host of medical problems. Sleep is a part of the rhythm of life and an absolute necessity for your body's recovery from the stresses of daily activities, injury, and illness.

WHY DO I REALLY NEED TO SLEEP?

Research has shown that drowsy people do worse in school and at work, tend to make poor decisions, and can cause accidents. One study showed that "sleep debts" accrue when nightly sleep totals six hours or fewer. The researchers found that those who routinely sleep six or fewer hours suffered from impaired cognitive abilities, including impaired calculation, memory, accuracy, and judgment. They also tend to think they've adjusted to a sleep debt, even though to avoid a sleep debt, the typical healthy adult needs an average of six to nine hours a night. Sleep plays an important role in energy homeostasis, a steady state of calorie intake and usage. New studies are showing a strong link between insufficient sleep, type 2

diabetes, and appetite control. As a result, sleep debt can have a harmful impact on carbohydrate metabolism, impaired glucose tolerance, and endocrine function. Women who sleep an average of five hours or less each night raise their risk of developing coronary heart disease compared with women who sleep eight hours.

HOW LONG AM I SUPPOSED TO SLEEP?

The amount of quality sleep each person needs varies and is influenced by your genetics, preference, age, previous sleep history, circadian rhythms, temperature, and medications. Of course, medical conditions such as sleep apnea and other sleep related disorders can affect the quality of your sleep. The general healthy range for sleep for adults is six to nine hours. Adolescents usually need more sleep, up to nine to nine and one half hours. The key is that you are not depriving yourself of sleep and you wake up feeling refreshed and don't feel sleepy during the day. To help you determine your sleep needs, go ahead and take the Sleep Quiz adapted from Peter Hudson Walters, PhD, CSCS, at Wheaton College, published in the *Strength and Conditioning Journal* in 2002, and see where you stand.

- Do you routinely fall asleep while reading a book, watching television, sitting in a movie theater, or riding as a passenger in a car for a trip less than an hour?
- Do you frequently fall asleep if you are in a quiet and dark environment for ten minutes?

- Does it take an alarm clock and several cups of coffee to get you going in the morning?
- Do you routinely have a hard time concentrating at work or always have a strong urge to fall asleep?
- Do you need "catch up" sleep on the weekends?
- Do you feel tired when you wake up?
- Do you frequently feel an overwhelming need to take naps during the day?

If you answered yes to at least two of these questions, then you are probably not getting enough sleep.

- Do you consistently sleep more than nine and one half hours per night?
- Do you feel lethargic or "slow" throughout the day?
- Do you sleep longer during times of stress, anxiety, or depression?

If you answered yes to at least two of these questions, then you may need less sleep.

The key is to find the optimal amount of sleep that allows you wake up feeling refreshed without the need for a grande latte to get you going.

Lessons from Life: Sleepwalking through Life

Lily, a 49-year-old attorney, wanted to get into great shape for her fiftieth birthday. She was exercising seven days a week in pursuit of her goal. She trained with weights three times a week for 30 minutes and then did cardio work for another 30 minutes, using either the stairclimber machine or elliptical trainer at her gym. On the other days she ran on the treadmill for 30 to 45 minutes at the gym. Even with all of this intense exercise she was having a difficult time losing body fat. Also she was starting to experience intermittent low back pain. Clearly, Lily was overtraining and there were some things out of balance in her lifestyle.

A closer evaluation of this high-powered attorney's lifestyle showed the following:

- She was sleeping five to six hours per night.

- She had enormous stress at work. She often worked through lunch and stayed late after everyone else was long gone.

- She sat in front of her computer at work for hours before getting up.

- After a long and hard day of work she trekked to her gym for her daily workout.

- She ate a very poor diet, often skipping breakfast and lunch and having chips, candy and soda in the late afternoon.

- She barely had time for her husband and two children due to her long day at work.

The following recommendations were made to Lily:

1 Increase her sleep to seven to eight hours per night.

2 See a physical therapist for her lower back pain. In physical therapy, she learned pain-free weight training exercises and emphasized core stability exercises for the abdominals and back, followed by stretching and relaxation exercises using yoga or Tai Chi.

3 Take frequent short stretch breaks every 30 to 45 minutes. Consult with a dietitian to learn how to eat healthy and prepare wholesome meals for home and work.

Lily and her husband decided to convert a part of the den into a family exercise room. The money they would save from many years of gym membership would easily offset the purchase price of a treadmill, large exercise ball, exercise mat, exercise elastic band, and free weights. She also cross trained by either walking outdoors at the local high school track, going for a hike near her home, or taking a bike ride in the neighborhood with her family. And she made it a habit to leave the office earlier so that she could spend quality time with her family.

After two months of incorporating these suggestions she reported feeling better and having more energy. Lily also lost about ten pounds and her body felt firmer even though she was exercising less. Finally, she noted that she had a more rewarding relationship with her husband and two children. Now meal preparation and exercise was becoming more of a family affair.

··

HOW CAN I IMPROVE MY SLEEP?

Since you spend about one third of your life sleeping, it's best to know how to get the most out of your night's sleep for optimal recovery and recharging. Maybe Benjamin Franklin was right when he said: "Early to bed and early to rise, makes a man healthy, wealthy, and wise." Here are some guidelines on getting a good night's sleep:

- Identify the amount of sleep you need to awaken feeling refreshed.

- Establish a regular bedtime and wake-up time and adhere to these times consistently throughout the week.

- Use your bed only for sleep and sex in order to associate your bed with relaxation rather than other activities such watching television.

- Sleep in a quiet, dark, cool, and comfortable room.

- Use ear plugs if you are in a noisy environment.

- Go to bed relaxed and not stressed. Stretch and do yoga, Tai Chi, Qi Gong, or relaxation exercises.
- Use relaxing bedtime rituals such as listening to soft music or reading a book.
- Avoid overexertion or heavy exercise immediately before sleep. Intense exercise should take place in the late afternoon or early evening at the latest, especially if you have difficulty sleeping.
- If you have difficulty falling asleep, avoid watching the news or reading an exciting book in bed, as these may cause you extra stress when you should be winding down.
- If you find yourself worrying about the next day's activity, jot down your schedule, and then allow your mind to relax. The key is to slow down and approach bedtime with a clear head.
- Avoid stimulants such as caffeine found in coffee, soft drinks and chocolate, alcohol, or nicotine, especially after about 3:00 p.m.
- Don't drink so much fluid in the evening that you are constantly waking up to go to the bathroom.
- Don't go to sleep starving or on a very full stomach.
- Take a warm shower or bath before going to bed.
- Don't try to force yourself to sleep. If you can't fall asleep within 15 to 20 minutes, get up, do something that relaxes you, and then go back to bed.

For further tips on obtaining proper sleep, refer to the following organizations:

- American Academy of Sleep Medicine, www.aasmnet.org
- National Institutes of Health National Center on Sleep Disorders Research, www.nhlbi. nih.gov/about/ncsdr
- National Sleep Foundation web site www.sleepfoundation.org

See a physician about pain or other medical problems which prevent you from sleeping properly, such as sleep apnea (a condition during which people stop breathing during sleep, sometimes for a minute at a time and sometimes hundreds of times during the night), headaches, or temporomandibular disorder of the jaw muscles or joints associated with chronic facial pain. Your primary physician may refer you to a physician specializing in sleep disorders if they suspect you may have sleep apnea, chronic insomnia (difficulty sleeping), or another sleep related disorder. Also, always consult with your physician before taking over-the-counter sleeping aids. Ultimately you may be masking a medical problem or simply masking the need for more consistent and longer sleep.

HOW DO I SELECT THE RIGHT MATTRESS AND PILLOW?

Finding an optimal mattress will take some time. When you are in the store, lie down on a few beds for at least five to ten minutes to get a feel for the different features. If it doesn't feel comfortable in the store, then it most likely won't feel comfortable in your home. You need a new mattress if:

- You are waking up sore and stiff.
- You are having a difficult time sleeping.
- Your bed is not providing enough support for your body.
- Your bed is sagging in the middle or just looks and feels worn out.
- You can feel "lumps" in your bed.
- Your bed is leaking its contents.
- Your bed is approximately ten years old.

Inadequate pillows have been linked with headaches, neck and back pain, morning neck stiffness, snoring, and an inability to sleep comfortably. If you have any lower back pain or hip discomfort, try placing a pillow between your knees.

Most pillows last only three to ten years. That's a wide range, but the time varies according to the quality of the pillow and the actual wear and tear. In general, the pillow height should comfortably support the head and neck in a neutral position. The pillow should be under your head, but not your shoulders.

Reduce Your Stress

Stress can be defined as the gap between what you want and expect from a situation and what really happens! Stressful situations include discovering a bear on your path through the woods, having a car accident, having a fight with your husband or wife, or being startled by the yell of your friends at your surprise party. At the very least, stress can prevent you from recovering after regular exercise and can contribute to your feeling anxious and tired. It is well-known that uncontrolled stress can have a bad effect on your overall health. Some signs of stress may include irritability, nervousness, fast heartbeat, impulsive and compulsive behavior, inability to concentrate, anxiety, sweating, indigestion, headaches, pain, loss of or excessive appetite, alcohol or drug addictions, increased smoking, nail biting, verbal and physical fighting, difficulty sleeping, and muscle tension.

Research has shown that stress can lead to weight gain or eating disorders and can delay wound healing. Stress can trigger overeating and underexercising, and ultimately, weight gain. Fat tissue signaling pathways are disrupted by stress, sometimes causing body fat storage. Negative emotional stress such as anger, fear, anxiety, bereavement, and depression can trigger heart attacks. The key is to identify the specific controllable stressors in your life and learn to minimize and control them.

WHAT CAN I DO TO RELAX?

Pay attention to what stimuli cause you undue stress. Keep a mental list of the types of activities that make your blood boil and brainstorm ways to cope a little better. For example, if you experience stress while driving in gridlock traffic, consider using public transportation, joining a carpool, or listening to relaxing music or a book on tape in the car. Explore your realistic alternatives, then tackle your stressors one by one and learn to minimize and control them.

What creates stress for you may not affect someone else in the same way. Hans Selye,

Lessons From Life: Cell Phone Stress

Cathy, a 36-year-old real estate agent, was running herself ragged at a high-profile real estate agency. As one of the top sellers every month, the cell phone ran her life 24-7. Her phone rang while she was driving, shopping at a grocery store, waiting in line at the bank, exercising on the treadmill while at gym, and as she was heading to bed.

The final insult came one evening while she was out dining with her fiancé. As usual, her personal time was interrupted again by a business call. Fortunately, her future husband was very understanding, but she could see his patience wearing thin with the constant barrage of calls. She realized that when you make yourself available to everyone at all hours, people will call you at all hours. She wanted to start her marriage on the right foot. She made a personal commitment to limit her time on the cell phone to business hours and for emergency use after work. She forwarded all her calls to her voice mail and checked them only during business hours.

A month later, Cathy realized her stress level had dramatically lessened and that her sleep had also improved. By setting boundaries with her work life, she was getting to bed earlier and sleeping more restfully, getting more and better quality sleep. Now, she can relax while walking and taking a Pilates class because her cell phone is turned off. Needless to say, her fiancé is happy that she no longer jumps out of her skin every time the phone rings.

MD, PhD, an endocrinologist who coined the term "stress" and wrote the groundbreaking book, *The Physiology and Pathology of Exposure to Stress,* in 1950, stated that "activity and rest must be judiciously balanced, and every person has his own characteristic requirements for rest and activity." Selye also said "the best way to avoid harmful stress is to select an environment (wife/husband/partner, boss, and friends) which is in line with your innate preferences—to find an activity which you like and respect. Only then can you eliminate the need for frustrating constant re-adaptation that is the major cause of distress." He also said "as long as man's pattern of behavior does not hurt others, he should live the life that is most natural to him." Of course, this is all easier said than done, but it is feasible to examine your life for activities that bring you happiness and peace and find ways to do these things a little more often.

The way a person handles stress appears to be more important than the stress itself. For instance, one person may perceive a particular situation as a stressful event and another person may perceive it as a challenge to rise to the occasion. The key is to identify what stressors cause you to react negatively and explore manageable solutions. Here are a few ideas on how to relax and reduce your stress levels (some of these will require long-term work but some you can put into practice right away):

Don't Live a "Type A Lifestyle": Are you always in a rush to get things done? Do you get impatient waiting in line? Instead, use that time wisely to take a mental break and relax. Try not to multi-task. Stop and focus on one task at a time and you'll find that you do it well.

Eat Right: Proper nourishment can have a positive influence on your mood and mental state. Registered dietitian Elizabeth Somer, RD, outlines the connection between food and your mental state in her book *Food & Mood*. The nutrition diaries in Part II will help you create an easy and healthy food plan.

Exercise: Physical activity can have a positive influence on your mood and mental state. Swimming and walking are gentle and relaxing forms of exercise. The activity maps in Part II will show you how to exercise safely and effectively.

Avoid Financial Problems: Stay out of unnecessary debt and spend within your means. Many resources, including books, online tools, and nonprofit organizations, are available if you need help learning how to set and maintain a budget.

Work at Having Good Family Relationships: Having a good relationship with your family goes a long way towards reducing and preventing stress. Of course, this is not something that you can accomplish overnight, but you can control how you react to stress from family members.

Get Variety in Life: Use variety in your exercises by cross training and get variety in the foods you eat. Occasionally try new experiences in life such as going to the opera, theater, or a ball game.

Pamper Yourself: Take a warm shower or bath, get a massage, or go to a spa for a manicure, facial, or other beauty treatments. (Men can do this, too!)

Gaze into the Distance: Focusing your eyes on far away pleasant scenery allows your body and mind to relax. Try star gazing, watching a sunset, looking at boats on water, watching birds fly. At work, look out your office window periodically and eat lunch outside. Go for walks in a park or mountain trail.

Be Around Wildlife: Play with your cat or dog. Watch and listen to birds. Get a pet turtle or fish aquarium to experience the slower side of life.

Laugh More: Laughing may help reduce stress and pain. Read the comics in the newspaper; watch a funny movie or television show.

Practice Positive Self Talk: You may think it's a little silly, but talking to yourself can put you in a positive mindset. Speak aloud phrases such as "I feel great today," "Today is going to be a great day at work," "My weekend is going to be fun." We're not suggesting that you ignore reality and not express any other emotions. The key is not

Battle Inflammation

Inflammation is your body's immune response against disease-causing microbes. It can be described as a nearly imperceptible internal swelling of tissues. It's how you fight infection, and once healing begins, inflammation stops. When inflammation gets out of control and continues on without a healing phase, it is chronic and can be responsible for a host of diseases including heart disease, stroke, and arthritis. It's hard to pinpoint, but one way to know if you have chronic inflammation is to ask for a blood test for C-reactive protein (CRP). This test is commonly performed to determine your risk for a heart attack.

We can make choices that greatly affect how our body handles inflammation. Certain foods can reduce inflammation by continuously supplying our body with compounds and nutrients that halt this immune response. Exercise regulates inflammatory markers helping alleviate inflammation and it helps to build muscle to support joints suffering from inflammation. Smoke is an irritant that will stimulate increased secretion of mucus. The inflammatory response from smoking can cause chronic obstructive pulmonary disease. Here's how you can help yourself:

- Eat more foods rich in omega-3 fatty acids such as flaxseeds and flaxseed oil, walnuts, and fish.
- Eat more foods rich in vitamin C such as strawberries, oranges, and red peppers.
- Eat more foods rich in vitamin E such as nuts and vegetable-based oils.
- Eat less saturated fat.
- Reduce body fat.
- Exercise regularly.
- Don't smoke.

to get trapped in a one-dimensional mind frame where everything in life is negative. **Use Positive Mental Imagery:** Close your eyes and visualize yourself accomplishing a goal or task. Imagine yourself getting over an obstacle or coming outside of the other end of the tunnel regarding a particular problem you are trying to tackle.

See a Medical Professional: If you have uncontrolled stress, then go see your physician. Your physician may recommend that you see a specialist, counselor or therapist to help you get back on the right track.

ARE THERE SPECIFIC TECHNIQUES I CAN USE TO RELAX?

In addition to the simple tips we've given you above, there are many formal relaxation techniques that you can use to relax from daily stresses, including yoga, Tai Chi, Qi Gong, the Alexander Technique, the Feldenkrais Method, and Jacobsen's Progressive Muscle Relaxation. These relaxation techniques can also be performed throughout the day at work or while traveling. See Resources and Further Readings on page 284 for more information about these relaxation techniques.

At the core of most of these techniques is some form of diaphragmatic breathing. Your breathing indicates how hard you are exerting yourself. Breathing patterns can also vary according to how relaxed or stressed you are. Sometimes when people are nervous, they breathe shallowly, with only their chest and shoulders moving with their breath. This excess muscle tension in the shoulders can lead to tightening of muscles in the neck and also throughout the body. Being able to control your breathing is one way of gaining control of your body's ability to relax.

Of course, you will still use chest breathing when you are exercising vigorously or running up the stairs to avoid being late for a meeting. But when you want to relax or ease anxiety, the key is to use a slower and deeper breathing technique, diaphragmatic breathing. This exercise will show you how it works.

Form: Your diaphragm is a dome-shaped muscle that sits on the bottom part of your lungs. Lie on your back in a quiet and dark room with a pillow under your knees and your eyes closed. Next, begin to breathe in and out through your nose (or through pursed lips if your nose has too much congestion). When you breathe in through your nose, your diaphragm moves down to allow your lungs to fill up with air. Of course, as your diaphragm moves down-

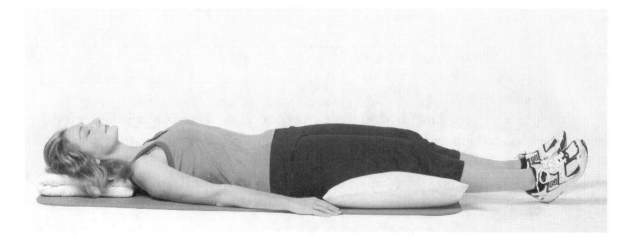

ward, it naturally causes your abdomen to expand slightly. Then when you breathe out, your diaphragm moves back upward into the chest, and your abdomen slowly sinks back down.

Other than the breathing pattern, you can also focus on the position of your jaw and tongue to increase your relaxation. For this part, start by assuming a relaxed jaw position. This is where the tip of your tongue is placed very lightly on the roof of your mouth, your lips are touching very lightly, and your teeth are not touching. This is called the N-Position because this is where your tongue would go when you are pronouncing the letter "n." Try saying the letter "n" out loud a couple of times and you'll quickly find the position. Practice this relaxed position throughout the day, especially if you suffer from nighttime teeth grinding or clenching.

Frequency: Do for 1 to 5 minutes. Keep in mind that one slow breath in and out is about 5 to 10 seconds. So 1 minute of breathing in this slow controlled manner would be about 6 to 12 breaths if you would rather count breaths. Counting breaths often works best for shorter relaxation breaks (ranging from 15 to 60 seconds). For longer periods, you may want to set a timer so you can totally relax. As you get used to the sensation (after several weeks or months of regular relaxation practice), you may find that you no longer need to count breaths or use a timer, and you can just go as long as your body needs to get the relaxation effect.

Chapter 2

Your Anti-Aging Exercise Basics

Fight Aging with Exercise

Your muscle mass takes a turn for the worse around age 50. Unless you exercise regularly, you lose one percent of your total muscle every single year due to a process known as sarcopenia. It doesn't sound like much, but if you choose a lifetime of inactivity, you'll have lost nearly 30% of your muscle by the time you reach 80 years old. Pair that with 20 added pounds of fat and you could very easily lose your ability to move about with ease, live independently, and care for your own needs.

Some normal physiological changes you can expect with age include a decline in cardiac output, renal function, maximal oxygen uptake (VO_2 max), and lung volume. Bone mass peaks by age 30, although you can maintain your current bone mass and prevent further loss through regular weight-bearing exercise and adequate nutrition. Your calorie-burning engine, your metabolism or BMR (basal metabolic rate), decreases by 5% per decade, and this is a culprit in fat gain later in life. While you're still a young adult, you're progressively losing flexibility, joint structures deteriorate, and your collagen fibers degenerate. But there's an alternative to losing ground physically as you age. And that alternative is exercise. Your body takes up the slack, and these changes do not limit your capacity to exercise nor do they limit your ability to benefit from exercise! And age doesn't affect your trainability.

There's no question that regular activity can help you regain some youthfulness and boost your quality of life. It benefits your mind by enhancing your ability to learn and improving your mood, it improves your glucose tolerance, blood cholesterol levels, blood pressure, and arthritis symptoms and, in turn, increases your life expectancy. Regular exercise enables you to retain much better cardiovascular functioning than your sedentary peers.

There are many reasons why people become inactive. When we have an injury or pain, we're often encouraged to take it easy. Poor weather conditions, pollution, and fears about safety keep people indoors and sedentary. But getting moving doesn't mean that you have to venture out of your comfort zone. Our program is not complicated, you can choose your venue, and we'll guide you through the transitions to push your limits gradually, safely, and easily using exercise guidelines from the American College of Sports Medicine (ACSM), an organization that promotes physical activity for people of all ages and sets the standard for exercise safety based on testing and current research.

The Perfect Triangle Prescription

We recommend a three-sided approach to your anti-aging fitness prescription. Think of a triangle with sides of equal length. They're all part of the shape, and one side is just as important as another to keep the shape. Your exercise prescription principles keep your shape by including three sides: strength, aerobic, and stretching. In as little as 30 minutes a day, you can be on your way.

Strength: Preserve your precious muscle mass by working your muscles against a resistance. The resistance will vary according to your fitness level. You can use your own body

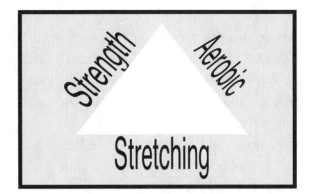

weight, a resistance band, a plate-loading variable resistance machine, such as Cybex or Nautilus, or dumbbells.

Aerobic: Choose from walking, biking, swimming, dance, and sports to get your heart rate elevated for cardio-respiratory (heart and lungs) benefit.

Stretching: Improve your flexibility and range of motion with two different types of stretches, static stretches and dynamic stretches. Static stretches involve taking a stretching exercise to a gentle end limit and holding that position for a period of time such as the ones we outline in this book. Dynamic stretching involves moving your body slowly and gradually increasing your range of movement such as when you perform yoga, Tai Chi or Qi Gong. Both types of stretches are beneficial to help loosen and prevent stiffness in muscles and joints. You can gauge where to begin based on what feels best to you.

In addition to strength, cardio-respiratory fitness, and flexibility, it's important for us to pay attention to our balance as we get older. A fall at any age can mean broken bones or an injury but this becomes more of a concern as we age since healing tends to be slower and the bones can be more brittle. Keeping your body flexible, strong, and in shape can help reduce your chances of falling, and many of the aerobic and strength-training exercises will also naturally force you to work on your balance. But doing specific balance exercises is also a good idea, and you'll find those incorporated into your Eight-Week Anti-Aging Fitness Prescription.

The eight-week program is designed for those of you who are in generally good health but haven't been exercising consistently in awhile (or ever). Even if you already do exercise regularly (good for you!), you'll find that the program is a helpful, easy, and effective way to fit in all the elements of fitness that you need to stay strong and healthy as you get older. We highly recommend that you check with your physician before engaging in the exercises outlined in this book. You should consider working with a physical therapist to help you modify the exercises according to your medical restrictions or limitations—if you've had hip, knee, shoulder or back surgery, for instance, or suffer from osteoporosis, high blood pressure, diabetes, or arthritis. For general fitness purposes, you should consider working with a qualified fitness professional or teacher of a particular method (such as yoga or Tai Chi) to ensure safety and proper instruction.

We are replacing the old and outdated philosophy of "no pain, no gain" with the "train without pain" philosophy. Remember, safety first.

Which Weigh to Anti-Aging?

In addition to keeping you flexible and functional, exercise, together with diet, helps you maintain a healthy weight—in itself an important arbiter of overall health. As you age, your fat mass increases and muscle mass decreases. As little as ten pounds of extra fat weight is connected to many diseases including type 2 diabetes, hypertension, elevated blood cholesterol, many types of cancer, and arthritis, to name just a few. A lifetime of little exercise and eating a few extra calories will catch up with you in the form of extra pounds. Most people report watching the pounds creep up slightly year by year, and suddenly it becomes a problem when years later, they have 20 pounds or more to lose. Shedding extra pounds before they start to accumulate is much easier to manage. Don't become the woe-is-me-when-did-all-this-weight-pile-on-me-I-need-to-lose-20-pounds-by-Friday monster. Some tips to keep the scale pointing in the right direction:

- Exercise and watch your calorie consumption.
- Weigh yourself regularly. If you're trying to lose weight, weigh yourself once a week, at the same time of day, and preferably without clothes.
- Include three servings of fruits and three servings of vegetables in your eating plan every day. The water and fiber will fill you up and your calorie intake will generally be lower.

Find a Certified Personal Trainer, Dietitian, or Physical Therapist

There are many organizations that certify personal fitness trainers. Two of the top organizations are the American College of Sports Medicine (ACSM) and the National Strength and Conditioning Association (NSCA). To find an ACSM certified trainer go to the ACSM's *Pro Finder* database at www.acsm.org. For a NSCA certified trainer go to the NSCA's *Find A Trainer* database at www.nsca-lift.org.

A registered dietitian (RD) is a health care professional who has studied nutrition at an American Dietetic Association (ADA)-approved college program and passed an exam for licensure with the ADA and, in many cases, the state. The ADA is the national professional organization representing registered dietitians. To find an RD or licensed nutritionist (who do basically the same job) in your area use the ADA's *Find A Nutrition Professional* database at www.eatright.org.

Physical therapists (PT) are health care professionals who have studied physical therapy at an American Physical Therapy Association (APTA)–approved college program and passed a national exam for licensure and fulfilled state license requirements to practice in that state. The PT diagnoses and treats people of all ages who have medical problems or other health related conditions that limit their abilities to move and perform functional activities in their daily lives. The APTA is the national professional organization representing physical therapists. To find a licensed PT in your area use the APTA's *Find A PT* database at www.apta.org.

- If you're not an exerciser, start slow and ease your new habit into your lifestyle.
- Determine your calorie needs using the "How many calories do you need?" formula on page 27.
- Measure your waist and have your body fat percentage tested (we'll tell you more about this in the next section).

- Keep on tracking. Use a food log, exercise log, track your weight once a week and your waist measurement and body fat percentage about every three months.

START HERE FOR WEIGHT LOSS

If you need to drop weight, it's a good idea to start with an assessment of your fat mass. The best indicator of this is your body fat percentage. Find a certified personal trainer to measure your body fat percentage. You can contact your local health club, university or hospital to see if they perform these tests. Try not to obsess about this measurement; it should be a marker of your progress, not a program-ending curse when you don't get the results you want.

The range for acceptable body fat percentages may seem broad, but this is to allow for athletes at the lower end of the spectrum. Don't shoot for body fat below the lowest numbers; body fat is good for some things! Your body fat plays a role with insulation against cold temperatures, nerve conduction, and cushioning between organs. The *American College of Sports Medicine's Resource Manual for Guidelines for Exercise Testing and Prescription* states that although there are no established norms for percent body fat, textbook authors and researchers propose the following guidelines.

- 34 years and younger: 8 to 22% for men and 20 to 35% for women
- 35 to 55 years old: 10 to 25% for men and 23 to 38% for women
- 56 years and older: 10 to 25% for men and 25 to 38% for women

Vivian H. Heyward, PhD, professor at the University of New Mexico, outlines the following ranges for obesity in her textbook *Advanced Fitness Assessment and Exercise Prescription*:

- 18 to 34 years old: 22% or higher for men; 35% or higher for women
- 35 to 55 years old: 25% or higher for men; 38% or higher for women
- 56 years and older: 23% or higher for men; 35% or higher for women

Studies have shown that your waist size can be used to help predict risk of heart disease, stroke, and type 2 diabetes. You may have heard of people having an apple shape (waist fat) or a pear shape (hip and thigh fat). Some studies have found that abdominal fat leads to more health problems such as increased risk of heart disease and diabetes.

For your waist size assessment, measure your waist in a standing position with a tape measure over the skin at your belly button level. In order to lower your risk of diabetes and heart disease, some researchers have suggested keeping your waist measurement 40 inches or less for men and 35 inches or less for women. Other studies recommend 35 inches or less for men and 31 inches or less for women. Either way, the goal is to avoid excess girth in your midsection and to reduce your body fat to help prevent these diseases and to keep you mobile as you age.

BODY MASS INDEX (BMI)

If you want to determine a healthy weight range for yourself, use the "normal" section of the BMI chart for a guideline. The BMI is a measure of body fat based only on height and weight. If you have a lower body fat percentage and a lot of muscle mass, your weight could be at the high end of the normal weight range or beyond, and this is normal and healthy for you. If you have a high body fat percentage and not much muscle mass, you can rely on the BMI guidelines more closely. Check out the BMI chart on page 26, and use this chart to identify your weight status.

How Many Calories Do You Need?

Get out your calculators. Here is an easy, accurate formula for determining your calorie needs. Keep in mind that for the very best results, you must be honest about your consistent daily activity level. Refer to the chart on page 27 to choose this number first, and then tackle the rest of the formula below. Be patient, and check your math. It's very important to know what your targeted calorie intake should be.

Based on this activity level, the following formula will give you the total number of calories that you need per day to maintain your current weight (number 7). If you want to lose weight, continue through the formula and complete number 8, and if you want to gain weight, skip 8, and complete through number 9.

The nutrition diaries in Part II give you a delicious 1600 calories every day, while the activity maps keep you moving to burn more calories. See the Mix 'N Match Anti-Aging Meal Plan on page 160 for nutritionally balanced options to adjust the calories in your meal plan as needed.

Calories Burned During Activity and Exercise

Now that you know how many calories you need, it's useful to know how many calories you burn with each activity you do. Before using the following calorie chart, choose the exercises that match your interests and abilities. These may not be the biggest calorie burners but if they're suited for you, then you're more likely to stick with them. All activity has its place and can be beneficial no matter how small the amount of calories burned. Variety will help prevent muscle imbalances, overuse injuries, and overtraining. It's the spice of life and makes activity more fun!

Body Mass Index Table

	Normal						Overweight					Obese																			Extreme Obesity					
BMI	19	20	21	22	23	24	25	26	27	28	29	30	31	32	33	34	35	36	37	38	39	40	41	42	43	44	45	46	47	48	49	50	51	52	53	54
Height (inches)																			**Body Weight (pounds)**																	
58	91	96	100	105	110	115	119	124	129	134	138	143	148	153	158	162	167	172	177	181	186	191	196	201	205	210	215	220	224	229	234	239	244	248	253	258
59	94	99	104	109	114	119	124	128	133	138	143	148	153	158	163	168	173	178	183	188	193	198	203	208	212	217	222	227	232	237	242	247	252	257	262	267
60	97	102	107	112	118	123	128	133	138	143	148	153	158	163	168	174	179	184	189	194	199	204	209	215	220	225	230	235	240	245	250	255	261	266	271	276
61	100	106	111	116	122	127	132	137	143	148	153	158	164	169	174	180	185	190	195	201	206	211	217	222	227	232	238	243	248	254	259	264	269	275	280	285
62	104	109	115	120	126	131	136	142	147	153	158	164	169	175	180	186	191	196	202	207	213	218	224	229	235	240	246	251	256	262	267	273	278	284	289	295
63	107	113	118	124	130	135	141	146	152	158	163	169	175	180	186	191	197	203	208	214	220	225	231	237	242	248	254	259	265	270	278	282	287	293	299	304
64	110	116	122	128	134	140	145	151	157	163	169	174	180	186	192	197	204	209	215	221	227	232	238	244	250	256	262	267	273	279	285	291	296	302	308	314
65	114	120	126	132	138	144	150	156	162	168	174	180	186	192	198	204	210	216	222	228	234	240	246	252	258	264	270	276	282	288	294	300	306	312	318	324
66	118	124	130	136	142	148	155	161	167	173	179	186	192	198	204	210	216	223	229	235	241	247	253	260	266	272	278	284	291	297	303	309	315	322	328	334
67	121	127	134	140	146	153	159	166	172	178	185	191	198	204	211	217	223	230	236	242	249	255	261	268	274	280	287	293	299	306	312	319	325	331	338	344
68	125	131	138	144	151	158	164	171	177	184	190	197	203	210	216	223	230	236	243	249	256	262	269	276	282	289	295	302	308	315	322	328	335	341	348	354
69	128	135	142	149	155	162	169	176	182	189	196	203	209	216	223	230	236	243	250	257	263	270	277	284	291	297	304	311	318	324	331	338	345	351	358	365
70	132	139	146	153	160	167	174	181	188	195	202	209	216	222	229	236	243	250	257	264	271	278	285	292	299	306	313	320	327	334	341	348	355	362	369	376
71	136	143	150	157	165	172	179	186	193	200	208	215	222	229	236	243	250	257	265	272	279	286	293	301	308	315	322	329	336	343	351	358	365	372	379	386
72	140	147	154	162	169	177	184	191	199	206	213	221	228	235	242	250	258	265	272	279	287	294	302	309	316	324	331	338	346	353	361	368	375	383	390	397
73	144	151	159	166	174	182	189	197	204	212	219	227	235	242	250	257	265	272	280	288	295	302	310	318	325	333	340	348	355	363	371	378	386	393	401	408
74	148	155	163	171	179	186	194	202	210	218	225	233	241	249	256	264	272	280	287	295	303	311	319	326	334	342	350	358	365	373	381	389	396	404	412	420
75	152	160	168	176	184	192	200	208	216	224	232	240	248	256	264	272	279	287	295	303	311	319	327	335	343	351	359	367	375	383	391	399	407	415	423	431
76	156	164	172	180	189	197	205	213	221	230	238	246	254	263	271	279	287	295	304	312	320	328	336	344	353	361	369	377	385	394	402	410	418	426	435	443

Source: Adapted from *Clinical Guidelines on the Identification, Evaluation, and Treatment of Overweight and Obesity in Adults: The Evidence Report.*

What describes your everyday activity level? (Choose just one activity.)

	Brisk Walking or Golfing Without a Cart or Swimming	Cycling or Aerobic Dancing Exercise (floorstyle aerobics)	Jogging	Activity Level	
				Women	Men
sedentary	Less than 30 minutes	Less than 22 minutes	Less than 11 minutes	1.0	1.0
low active	30 minutes	22 minutes	11 minutes	1.14	1.12
active	1 3/4 hours	1 1/3 hours	40 minutes	1.27	1.27
very active	4 1/4 hours	3 hours	1 1/2 hours	1.45	1.54

How many calories do you need?

Women	Men
1. Multiply your age by 7.31 _____ (A)	1. Multiply your age by 9.72 _____ (A)
2. Subtract A from 387 _____ (B)	2. Subtract A from 864 _____ (B)
3. Multiply your weight (in pounds) by 4.95 _____ (C)	3. Multiply your weight (in pounds) by 6.46 _____ (C)
4. Multiply your height (in inches) by 16.78 _____ (D)	4. Multiply your height (in inches) by 12.8 _____ (D)
5. Add C + D _____ (E)	5. Add C + D _____ (E)
6. Multiply E by your Activity Level _____ (F)	6. Multiply E by your Activity Level _____ (F)
7. Add B + F _____ This is your calorie target to maintain your weight!	7. Add B + F _____ This is your calorie target to maintain your weight!
8. If you want to lose weight, deduct 500 calories from your answer to number 7 to lose 1-2 pounds per week: _____	8. If you want to lose weight, deduct 500 calories from your answer to number 7 to lose 1-2 pounds per week: _____
9. If you want to gain weight, be sure to do strength building exercises to build some muscle weight and add 500 calories to your answer to number 7 to gain about 1 pound a week: _____	9. If you want to gain weight, be sure to do strength building exercises to build some muscle weight and add 500 calories to your answer to number 7 to gain about 1 pound a week: _____

Note that your calculation for B will be a negative number if you are a woman over 52 or a man over 88.

Reprinted with permission from Dietary Reference Intakes for Energy, Carbohydrate, Fiber, Fat, Fatty Acids, Cholesterol, Protein, and Amino Acids (Macronutrients) © 2005 by the National Academy of Sciences, courtesy of the National Academies Press, Washington, DC.

Approximate Calories Burned Per Hour

Activity	Sample Body Weight	
	130 lbs	180 lbs
Basketball (shooting baskets)	265	365
Basketball (playing a game)	470	650
Bicycling (stationary, 50 Watts, very light effort)	175	240
Calisthenics (light or moderate effort home exercises)	205	285
Gardening (general)	235	325
Golf (walking and pulling your golf clubs)	250	350
Hiking (cross country)	350	485
Jogging (general)	410	570
Mowing lawn (walking and using a hand mower)	350	490
Sitting-writing, desk work, typing	105	145
Skiing (downhill – light effort)	295	405
Sleeping	50	70
Stretching (mild)	145	200
Soccer (casual)	410	570
Softball	295	405
Swimming (leisurely, not lap swimming)	350	485
Swimming (freestyle lap swimming, light or moderate effort)	410	570
Tennis (singles)	470	650
Tai Chi	235	325
Walking (2.0 mph, level and firm surface, slow pace)	145	200
Walking (3.0 mph, level surface, moderate pace)	190	265
Walking (3.5 mph, level surface, brisk pace)	220	310
Weightlifting (free weight, plate loading variable resistance machines- light or moderate effort)	175	240
Weightlifting (free weight, plate loading variable resistance machines - vigorous effort)	350	490

Sources: 1) Ainsworth BE, Haskell WL, Whitt MC, et al. Compendium of physical activities: An update of activity codes and MET intensities. *Medicine and Science in Sports and Exercise.* 2000;32(9):S498-S516.

2) Ainsworth BE, Haskell WL, Leon AS, et al. Compendium of physical activities: Classification of energy costs of human physical activities. *Medicine and Science in Sports and Exercise.* 1993;25 (1):71-80.

Chapter 3

Your Warm-Up and Stretching Exercises

Warm-Up Program

Warming up allows your body to ease into an activity while a cool-down allows your body to ease out of an activity safely. A warm-up prepares your body for activity by increasing circulation, lubricating the joints, increasing tissue extensibility, and mentally preparing you to train or just move around comfortably. The cool-down period provides a gradual recovery for the heart muscle and all the other body systems. So doing warm-up and cool-down exercises can mean the difference between injury and safety.

What Equipment Do I Need?

Exercise mat: Use a well-cushioned and non-slip exercise mat, such as an Airex mat.

Pillow or towel: Use a small pillow or towel to support your head and neck.

How Long Should I Warm Up and Cool Down?

Your exercise session should begin and end with a 5- to 10-minute low-intensity, calisthenic activity (such as the Warm-Up Routine that follows) or with low-intensity walking or stationary bicycling. The amount of time you spend warming up and cooling down depends on the type of activity that you will be doing. If you are going for a walk, then 5 minutes of warm-up and cool-down will probably be enough, but a tennis match may require 5 to 10 minutes.

An alternative way for you to warm up and cool down may be to do some gentle yoga, Tai Chi, or Qi Gong. Another great way to cool down is to try diaphragmatic breathing after the activity session to relax and calm your muscles and mind.

WARM-UP EXERCISES

You can perform this following simple warm-up routine before workouts or in the morning to get yourself loose for the day.

March in Place

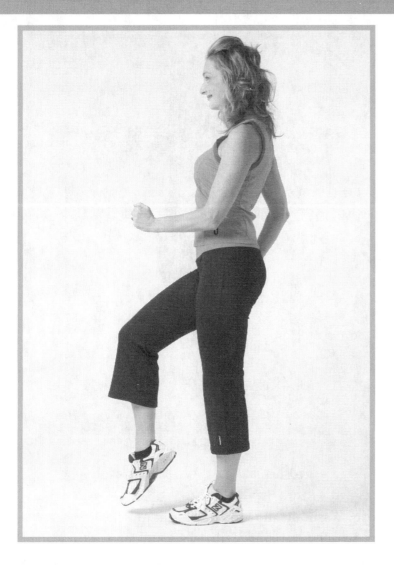

Purpose: Warm up the leg muscles.

Form: Start by standing with the legs hip width apart. Slowly bend your knees to lift your legs alternately to about hip height or as high as is comfortable. Begin slowly and progress to a brisk pace within your comfort zone.

Frequency: Do 10 to 50 repetitions (or reps for short) depending on your level of fitness.

Shake, Rattle and Roll

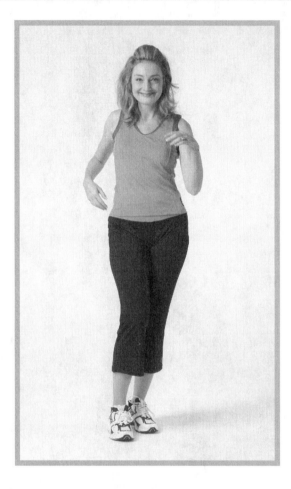

NOTE: If you work in front of a computer most of the day, perform this exercise at least every 20 to 50 minutes to keep your wrist and hands loose.

32

Purpose: Warm up and loosen the arm muscles.

Form: Start by standing with legs shoulder width apart. Begin by gently shaking your hands and arms. Then add a back–and–forth arm motion as if you were swinging your arms while walking. To get a better picture in your mind as to how this looks, think of how Olympic swimmers shake their arms before they start a race or how a cat shakes his paw when he's stuck it in some water.

Frequency: Shake, rattle and roll for 10 reps with each arm.

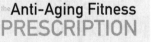

Trunk Rotations

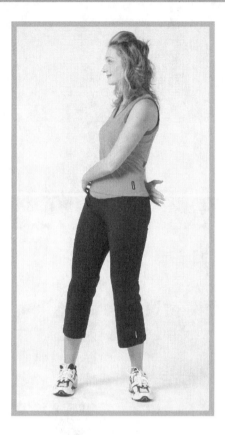

Purpose: Warm up the trunk and shoulder muscles.

Form: Start by standing with your legs shoulder width apart, trunk and head rotated slightly to the right. Your right hand should swing towards the left side of your lower back; your left hand, towards the right side of the front part of your hip. Slowly rotate your entire trunk to the left and let your arms unwind so that your trunk and head turns left. Your right hand ends up at the front of your left hip; your left hand, behind your right lower back. Perform this motion slowly and gently to loosen up your trunk and shoulders.

Frequency: Do 10 reps.

Lower Back Cat/Camel

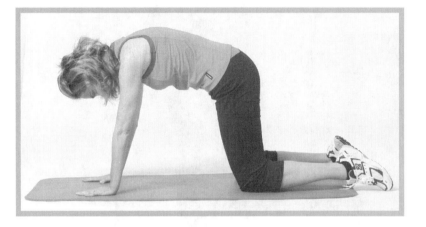

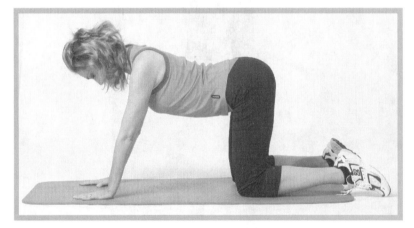

PRECAUTION: **Skip this exercise if it causes knee pain, wrist pain, or lower back pain. If you have osteoporosis, a back or neck injury, or had total knee or hip replacement surgery, then consult with your healthcare provider or your physical therapist before you try this exercise.**

34

Purpose: Warm up the lower back.

Form: Start on your hands and knees with your knees shoulder width apart. Slowly curl your lower back upward partially like an angry cat. Then arch your lower back downward partially like a dip in a roller-coaster. Keep your abdominal muscles relaxed and your head looking down, neck straight.

Frequency: Do 10 reps.

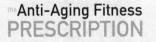

Heel Sits with Arms in Front

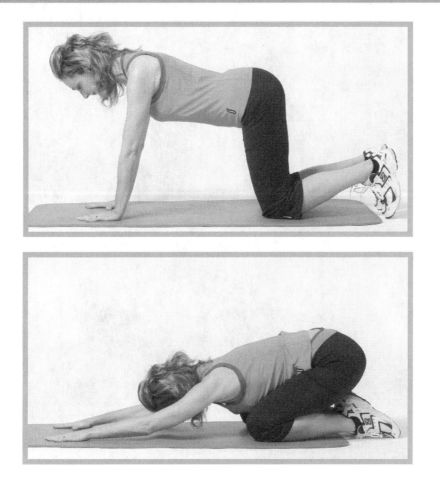

Purpose: Warm up the hips and middle of the lower back.

Form: Start on your hands and knees with your knees shoulder width apart. Place both hands in front of your body. Slowly sit back straight towards your heels and then return to the starting position. Keep your head in neutral by looking at the floor.

Frequency: Do 10 reps.

Heel Sits with Arms to Side

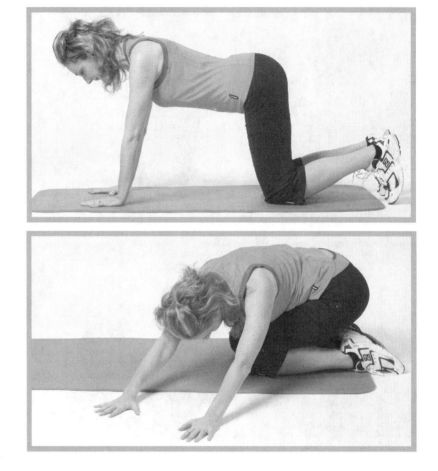

Purpose: Warm up the hips and sides of the lower back and torso.

Form: Start on your hands and knees with your knees shoulder width apart. Place both hands off to the sides of your body, as far as is comfortable. Slowly sit back on your heels and then return to the starting position for 10 reps. Now move your hands to the opposite side and repeat for another 10 reps. As you sit back towards your heels you will feel a stretch on the side of your back opposite your hands.

Frequency: Do 10 reps on each side.

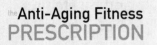

the **Anti-Aging Fitness**
PRESCRIPTION

Hip Windshield Wiper

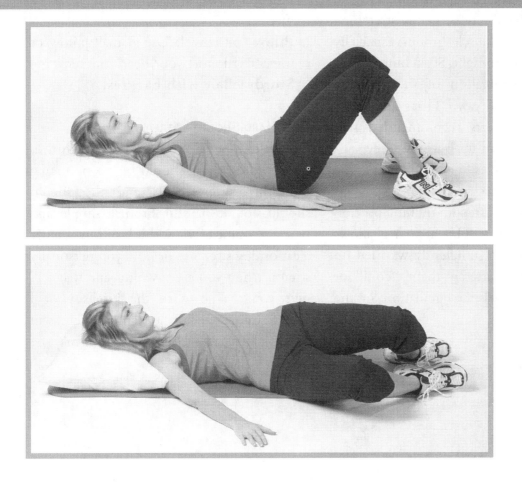

Purpose: Warm up the hips and lower back.

Form: Start by lying on your back with a pillow or towel under your head, knees bent and feet shoulder width apart. Slowly rotate your knees from side to side, keeping your knees together.

Frequency: Do 10 reps.

37

Chapter 3

Your Warm-Up and Stretching Exercises

Stretching Program

Flexibility gives your body the freedom to move and makes it long and lean. You can increase your flexibility by gently stretching all of your major muscle groups, especially the muscles that are tight. Stretching is simply a gentle elongation of the muscles. Think of when you yawn. That's stretching.

Previously, experts recommended that you stretch to warm up, but now they suggest that the muscles and tendons may be more responsive to stretching during or after the aerobic or strength training portion of a training routine. This approach allows your muscles to be sufficiently warmed up before trying to stretch them "cold" or without first increasing circulation in the area.

WHAT EQUIPMENT DO I NEED?

Exercise mat: Use a well-cushioned and non-slip exercise mat, such as an Airex mat.

Pillow or towel: Use a small pillow or towel to support your head and neck.

Sturdy chair with backrest

HOW HARD SHOULD I STRETCH?

Stretch to a position of mild discomfort. In other words, there should be no bouncing or jerking movements and the stretch should not be painful. From a simple and practical point of view, think of how gently a cat or dog stretches or how you personally stretch when you are yawning, and that will give you a clue as to the intensity of a stretch. Sport-specific stretching, such as in ballet, martial arts, or gymnastics, may be

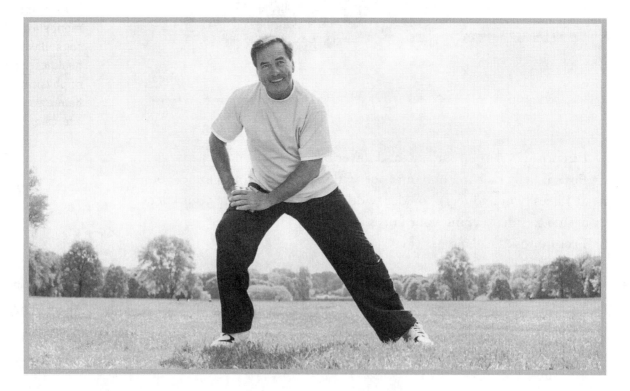

more aggressive because the goal of stretching for these sports is different.

How Long Should I Stretch?

Aim for 15 to 30 seconds for each stretch. A study in the journal *Physical Therapy* found that people aged 65 years or older may benefit from longer periods of hamstring stretching (60-second duration) to improve range of motion.

One way to measure the length of time you hold a stretch is to breathe slowly using the diaphragmatic technique for a certain number of breaths instead of counting the seconds. This may help you to relax more and you'll be able to meet the time requirement for stretching as well. For example, 30 seconds could be roughly 6 slow diaphragmatic breaths.

Aim for 1 to 3 sets for each stretch. From a practical standpoint, you could stretch for 1 set but perform the stretch several times a day.

How Often Should I Stretch?

It depends. You may need to stretch daily, or even several times per day, to attain specific goals and prevent muscle imbalances. And you should stretch whenever you are doing other types of exercise. Once again, watch how many times your cat or dog stretches during the day. They're stretching all over the place! Stretching throughout the day is a great way to prevent stiffness and muscle tension. If you don't otherwise need to stretch, though, aim for a minimum of 2 to 3 days per week.

Stretching Exercises

Do the following stretches after your exercise program.

Wrist Stretch

PRECAUTION: Avoid bending the wrists to excess range in either direction to prevent injury.

NOTE: If you work in front of a computer most of the day, perform this stretch at least every 20 to 50 minutes to keep your wrist and hands flexible.

40

Purpose: Stretch the forearm muscles on the palm and backhand side.

Form: Start in a sitting or standing position. The first part involves gently placing your palms together in a prayer position in front of your chest and holding. The second part involves hanging your arms straight by your sides and gently curling your wrists upwards and back towards your palms.

Frequency: Hold for 3 to 6 breaths (or 15 to 30 seconds) and repeat for 1 to 3 sets.

the **Anti-Aging Fitness**
PRESCRIPTION

Neck Stretches

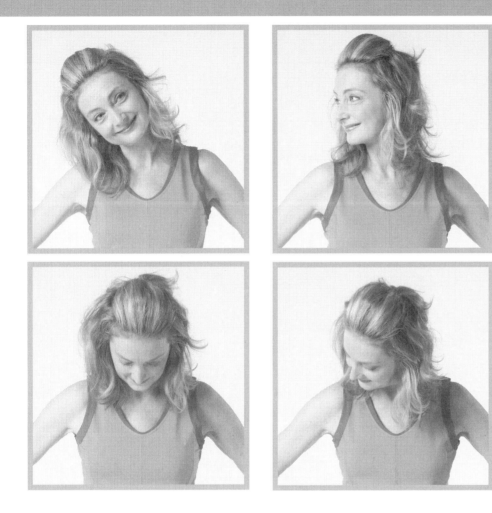

PRECAUTION: **Skip these exercises if they cause pain in the arms or shoulders.**

Purpose: Stretch the neck.

Form: Start in a sitting or standing position for all of the following stretches.

a) Neck Sidebend Stretch. Allow your head to move slowly toward your right ear. Allow gravity to provide the stretch. Then allow your head to move toward your left ear.

b) Neck Rotation Stretch. Slowly turn your head (as if you are shaking your head "no") toward your right shoulder comfortably, then your left shoulder.

c) Gentle Chin Nod Stretch. Slowly nod your head down toward your chest.

d) Look to Armpit. Slowly bend your neck diagonally down to look at your right armpit, then your left.

Frequency: Hold each stretch position for 1 to 2 breaths (or 5 to 10 seconds) and repeat for 1 to 3 sets.

Chapter 3

Your Warm-Up and Stretching Exercises

Hands Behind Back Stretch

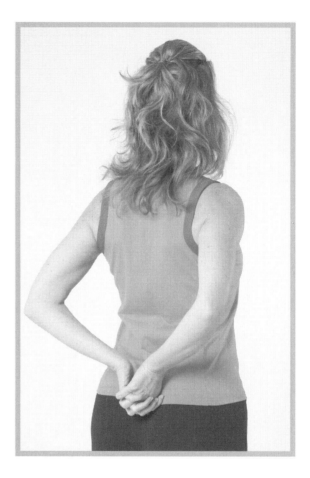

42

Purpose: Stretch the shoulder muscles.

Form: Start in a standing position. Place your hands behind your back, with your thumbs almost touching the bottom of your spine, and reach up towards your shoulder blades. Your elbows bend as you reach up your back.

Frequency: Hold for 3 to 6 breaths (or 15 to 30 seconds) and repeat for 1 to 3 sets.

Hands Behind Head Stretch

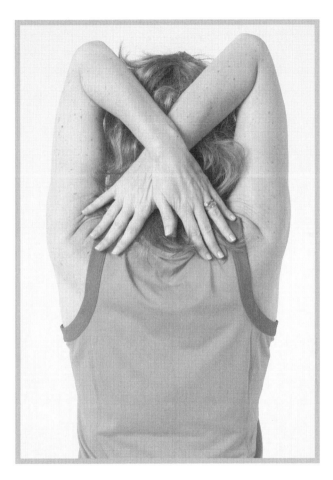

PRECAUTION: **Keep your head looking straight ahead and avoid rounding your shoulders forward to avoid straining your neck. Avoid this exercise if it causes pain or symptoms in the arms or shoulders.**

Purpose: Stretch the shoulder and triceps muscles.

Form: Start in a standing position. Place your hands behind your head and reach down towards the inner part of your shoulder blades. Your elbows bend as you reach down the back of your neck.

Frequency: Hold for 3 to 6 breaths (or 15 to 30 seconds) and repeat for 1 to 3 sets.

43

Yawn Stretch

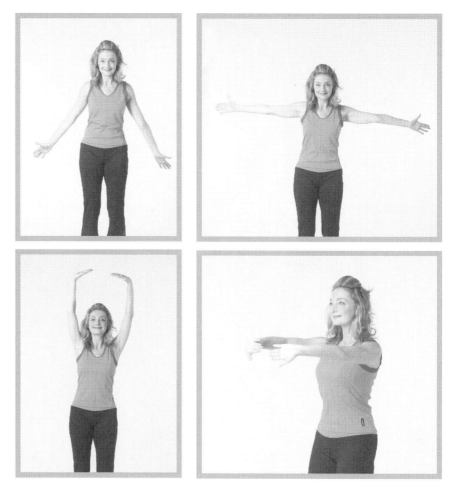

44

Purpose: Stretch the arms, chest, and back.

Form: Start in a standing position. Begin with your arms by your hips with your palms facing the floor. Then slowly raise the arms to shoulder height with the palms facing the side walls. Continue to slowly raise your arms to an overhead position with your palms facing the ceiling. Finally, lower your arms to the front of your body to chest height with palms facing towards the front wall.

Frequency: Hold each position for 1 breath (or 5 seconds) and repeat for 1 to 3 sets.

Look Over the Shoulder Stretch

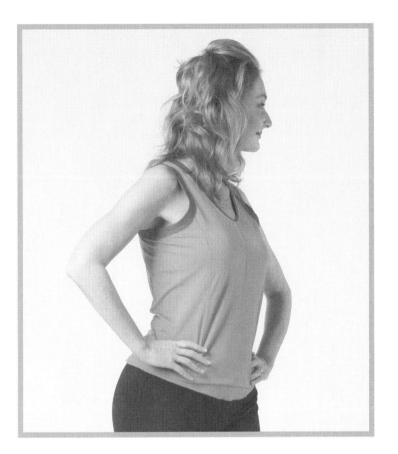

Purpose: Stretch the neck, shoulder, back, and hips.

Form: Start in a standing position with feet shoulder width apart. Place your hands on your hips. Slowly look over your left shoulder gently by turning your neck, shoulders, torso and hips and then hold. Repeat to the right side.

Frequency: Hold each position for 1 to 2 breaths (or 5 to 10 seconds) and repeat for 1 to 3 sets.

Calf Stretch

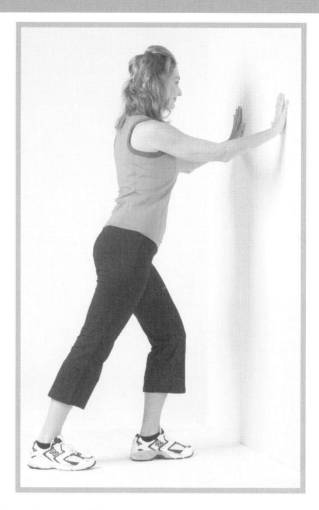

Purpose: Stretch the calf muscle.

Form: Stand facing a wall and place your hands on the wall at about shoulder height for stability and to maintain good posture. Place your right leg behind you with your foot pointed straight ahead and knee straight. Place your left leg in front of you with your knee in a bent position to support yourself. Now slowly lean your torso forward so you feel a stretch in your right belly of the calf muscle and in the heel cord. Repeat on the left side.

Frequency: Hold for 3 to 6 breaths (or 15 to 30 seconds) and repeat for 1 to 3 sets.

Hip Flexor Stretch

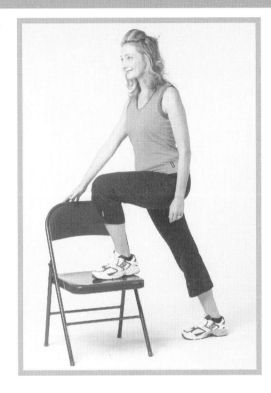

47

Purpose: Stretch the muscles in front of the hips and legs and also the calf.

Form: Start in standing position facing a chair with a backrest positioned sideways. Hold onto the back of the chair and place your left foot on a chair with your knee bent. Your right leg remains on the floor with your knee straight and foot pointed forward. Keep your back straight and then lean forward at your hips while putting most of your weight on the leg that is on the floor. You should feel the stretch in front of the right hip and right calf and slightly in the left calf. Use your hand on the backrest for stability and balance. Switch leg positions to stretch the left hip.

Frequency: Hold for 3 to 6 breaths (or 15 to 30 seconds) and repeat for 1 to 3 sets.

Hamstring Stretch

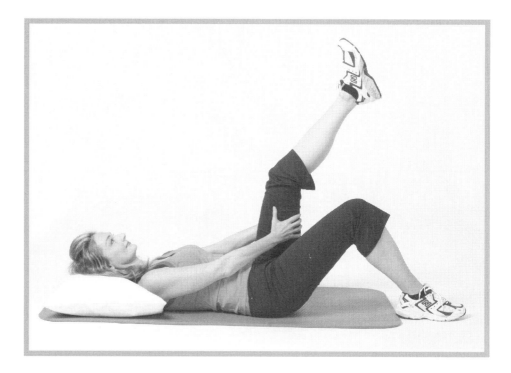

48

Purpose: Stretch the muscle on the back of the thigh.

Form: Start by lying on your back with a pillow under your head and both knees bent. Place one hand under your left knee and slowly straighten your left leg towards the ceiling as far as you can and hold in a comfortable position where you feel the stretch in the back of your thigh. From that position slowly move your foot toward you and away from you to further feel a stretch behind your knee and calf. Repeat on the right leg.

Frequency: Hold for 3 to 6 breaths (or 15 to 30 seconds) and repeat for 1 to 3 sets.

Quadriceps Stretch

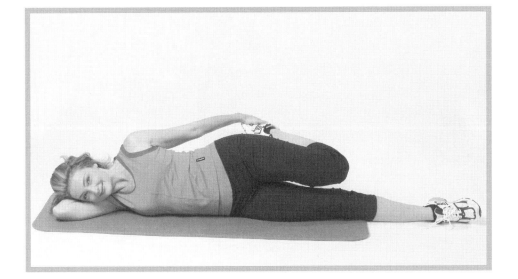

Purpose: Stretch the muscle on the front of the thigh.

Form: Start by lying on your right side with both of your knees slightly bent and your right arm under your head for support. Grasp your left ankle and pull towards your buttocks until you feel a stretch in the front of your left thigh. As you pull your left knee towards your buttock, also pull your left hip backwards to where it is aligned straight with your torso as if you are standing upright. Repeat on the right leg.

Frequency: Hold for 3 to 6 breaths (or 15 to 30 seconds) and repeat for 1 to 3 sets.

Inner Hip Stretch

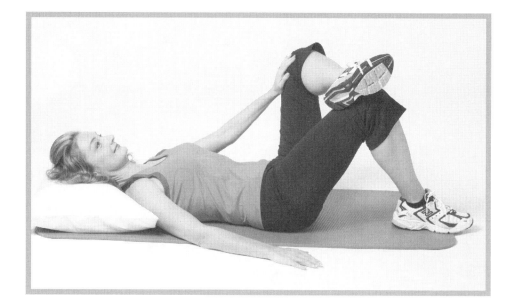

Purpose: Stretch the inner hip and thigh muscles.

Form: Start by lying on your back with a pillow or towel under your head, both knees bent, and your feet flat on the floor. Slowly bend your knee and hip so that your left heel rests on your right knee. Gently place your left hand on your left knee and apply a very gentle force away from you to stretch the left inner hip region. Repeat on the right leg.

Frequency: Hold for 3 to 6 breaths (or 15 to 30 seconds) and repeat for 1 to 3 sets.

Outer Hip Stretch

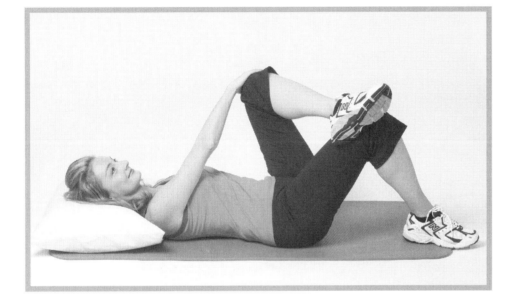

PRECAUTION: **Skip this stretch if this position causes pain in your hips or lower back. If you have osteoporosis, a back or neck injury, or had total knee or hip replacement surgery, then consult with your healthcare provider or physical therapist before you try this exercise.**

Purpose: Stretch the outer hip and thigh muscles.

Form: Start by lying on your back with a pillow or towel under your head, both knees bent, and your feet flat on the floor. Slowly bend your knee and hip so that your left heel rests on your right knee. Place your right hand on the outer part of your left knee. Gently pull your left knee toward your right shoulder to feel a stretch in your left buttocks. Repeat on the right leg.

Frequency: Hold for 3 to 6 breaths (or 15 to 30 seconds) and repeat for 1 to 3 sets.

51

Chapter 3

Your Warm-Up and Stretching Exercises

Chapter 4

Your Aerobic Exercise

Aerobic exercise gives your body the endurance to sustain activity. Cardio-respiratory fitness is the ability to perform large-muscle (in which large muscles such as the gluteus maximus and quadriceps muscles are engaged), dynamic, moderate- to-high-intensity exercise for prolonged periods. Your goal with doing aerobic exercise is to improve the ability of your heart and lungs to adapt and recover from stress and exercise.

Do you know someone who gets winded during short walks, such as retrieving the newspaper in the morning or walking across a parking lot into a store? As we age, cardiac output decreases and the lung tissue becomes less elastic causing a decrease in expiratory flow and lung volume. But this should not stop you from making gains with aerobic exercise! Your capacity to do aerobic exercise and your ability to benefit from exercise is not impaired with aging.

As we noted earlier, we follow American College of Sports Medicine (ACSM) recommendations for aerobic duration and intensity. This is simple and very safe. You may have seen various aerobic programs that focus upon getting your heart rate to a certain range. We prefer not to use these formulas because too many people focus so much on reaching their heart rate range or getting to a certain intensity on a bike or taking a certain amount of steps on a treadmill that they ignore how they feel. They may have a headache, knee pain, an upset stomach, or feel very fatigued, but may push themselves to the point of injury in order to reach their target. Exercise does not have to be complicated or painful for it to be effective! Target heart rates are not appropriate for everyone. We feel that using heart rate alone as a gauge of exercise intensity is not totally reliable. In

Part II, we'll introduce you to the OMNI RPE scale which is a formal way for you to gauge how hard you are working during exercise and activity. You'll also learn how to gauge your intensity level through our Self Monitoring Scale.

What Equipment Do I Need?

Walking shoes: See the section below for selecting a proper shoe

Pedometer (optional)

Treadmill (optional)

Recumbent bike (optional)

Note: If you are planning to equip a home gym, we recommend staying with the basics. A treadmill offers a basic weight bearing exercise; the recumbent bike offers an exercise that does not stress the joints and does not require balance. Other machines for the home do not have as much versatility. The elliptical machine, for instance, may cause an overuse problem in the hip; the stairclimber can do the same for the knees; and the aerobic rower can aggravate the low back. In a gym, you can cross-train between many types of machines and therefore minimize these types of overuse problems, but that's impractical in most homes.

What Is Considered Aerobic Exercise?

Walking, hiking, outdoor cycling, dancing, running, swimming, cross-country skiing, skating, rowing, and recreational endurance games (such as tennis, volleyball, basketball,

badminton, racquetball), certain types of martial arts are all considered aerobic exercise. You can also use aerobic exercise machines, such as stair climbers, cross-country skiers, rowers, upper body and lower body cycling machines, elliptical machines, or treadmills.

How Hard Should I Do Aerobic Exercise?

Aim for a pace hard enough to work up a sweat but one that allows you to talk with a friend without gasping for breath. Pay attention to how you feel. You shouldn't be totally breathless and fatigued and you shouldn't have pain, dizziness, or headache during or after the exercise session. Exercise should not be torture. After all, you're doing all this to feel better!

How Long Should I Do Aerobic Exercise?

Aim for 30 to 45 minutes of aerobic activity accumulated throughout the day. It's easy to start with walking. You can get up from your desk at work and do office errands, keep walking, and time yourself. Invest in a pedometer and challenge yourself to keep making more gains. You might want to start with short 5- to 10-minute bouts throughout the day or do a single 30- to 45-minute session with rests if you need them.

Walking is a safe way to be active. Most people can safely incorporate a walking program for 30 minutes on most days of the week. This can be a great start to improving your fitness level. A good surface to walk on is a relatively flat grass surface (like a park) or a rubberized track surface (like a college or high school track). If this is not available and your only choice is the mall or your neighborhood sidewalk, then a good pair of shoes is very important to help cushion the impact.

How Often Should I Do Aerobic Exercise?

Ideally, you should do some sort of aerobic exercise 3 to 5 times per week. However, 2 times per week may be needed initially to build up your endurance. If you're new to exercising, start out slow. You may be eager to see results from your new routine, but remember your days were full of other activities before you started exercising. You'll soon resent the time spent exercising and be more likely to abandon your new program. Move slowly, you won't even know the difference, and you'll be less likely to make excuses to skip workouts. So hold your horses to make your new habit stick!

Are There Things I Should Avoid When Doing Aerobic Exercises?

Avoid Bleacher or Stadium Step Running or Walking

Visit a college or high school track or football stadium on the weekend, and you will often see people walking or running up and down the stadium steps. Most people aren't aware of the potentially harmful effects on the knee, ankle, hip, and lower back joints when they do this type of exercise.

Osteoarthritis is the most common degenerative joint disease in 60% of adults over 50 years of age, and the knee is the most commonly affected joint. Overloading the hip and knee joints, with activities such as walking or running stadium stairs, may lead to cartilage breakdown or failure of other structures (such as ligaments). If you are significantly overweight, you are at even greater risk for overdoing exercise and experiencing injury. It's definitely not worthwhile to court an injury, one that can really affect your lifelong mobility, just to burn more calories. The key is to go slow and progress in smaller increments and the weight will come off gradually. Your goal should be long-term success and not what you can lose in a couple of weeks.

Avoid Walking, Running, or Doing Sports with Ankle or Hand Weights

Holding light weights, ranging from 1 to 3 pounds, while walking can increase the intensity of aerobic exercise. However, this common practice may lead to shoulder, elbow, and wrist overuse injuries, as well as back and neck strain and headaches. Placing weights on the ankles, in an attempt to develop leg strength, may lead to hip and back problems.

We'd all like to multi-task, but using cuff weights in this fashion may lead to overuse injuries in your lower back, hip, or shoulder. Unless you are in a controlled class being monitored by trained professionals (some step classes, for instance, use weights), the safer alternative is to train your lower and upper body muscles individually for strength and perform your aerobic program without the ankle or hand weights. If your goal is to run faster or jump higher, then you should do speed training and jump-specific training.

How Do I Select Good Shoes For My Workouts?

It is very important to select a proper shoe for your exercise program, daily activities, work, and sports. Athletic shoes are designed to protect certain areas of your feet that encounter the most stress during the activity. Proper athletic shoes can also help reduce the harmful forces transmitted to the knees, hips and spine. Ideally, you'll need a specialized shoe for running, walking, aerobics classes (including floor or step routines), or court sports (such as tennis, volleyball, and basketball). If you have any specific foot concerns, then consult with a podiatrist, physical therapist, or physician.

After 300 to 400 miles, your shoes have lost about half their cushioning. However, mileage alone will not tell someone when they should replace worn-out shoes. There are other factors that can determine the life of your shoe: the name brand of the shoe; the conditions the shoe is worn under (if you live in a humid climate, for instance, your shoes may wear out faster); your weight; and whether you are a pronator

(your feet roll in and flatten at the arch area) or a supinator (you put weight on the outsides of your foot). As a general guide, you need new shoes when:

- your old shoes lean inward or outward (as you look at the shoes from the back)
- the glue holding the shoe together is beginning to come apart
- the shoe shows excess wear on the edges of the sole
- you have logged approximately 500 miles in them
- you notice pain and discomfort in your feet, ankles, knees, or legs.

When shopping, take the socks and orthotics (if applicable) that you will wear during the sport or workout. Find a good store with knowledgeable salespeople that will address your needs. Shop during the day, if you can; you're more likely to find full-time staff then, who are usually more informed about the products. Have both feet measured for length and width every time you buy a new shoe, since foot size changes as we age and shoe size may vary among different name brands. Buy the shoe size that fits the longer and/or wider foot. To measure your feet properly:

- Generally, for a high-arched foot, look for cushioned shoes (a curved, flexible last). For a flat foot, look for a motion control shoe (medial posts, a straight last, and a firm heel cup). For a normal foot, look for a stability shoe (semi-curved last). A shoe last is the solid from around which a shoe is molded. The fit of a shoe depends on the design, shape and volume of the shoe last.

- Lace shoes properly while testing.
- Make sure there is at least one thumb's width of space (approximately ½ inch) from the longest toe to the end of the toebox. The shoe should be long enough so that you can wiggle all your toes and they can fully extend without being cramped.
- The width of the shoe should match the widest part of the foot and allow for movement of the toes and spreading of the foot. Your shoes may be too tight if your toenails turn black from rubbing, your feet cramp, your feet fall asleep and/or you get calluses and blisters between your toes.
- Make sure the heel collar is soft and does not put too much pressure on the Achilles tendon.
- Try to approximate the conditions the shoes will be worn under (walking, running, jumping or side-to-side movement as in tennis and basketball). Also, try the shoes on a non-carpeted area to feel them on a hard surface.

Don't let slick advertising hook you to one name brand. Try on various brands and pick the one that feels the best and gives you all the features you need. You get what you pay for, so expect to spend some money for quality shoes. But remember, the feel and fit of your shoes are the most important, not the appearance. A proper fitting shoe will be comfortable from the moment you step in it and will fit well from the first day. Don't expect to "break in" an uncomfortable shoe.

Carefully inspect and feel the shoes for defects that may have been missed at the manufacturer. Check to see if the shoe is glued together properly and air and gel pockets are inflated evenly.

Chapter 5

Your Strength Training and Balance Exercises

Strength training (also known as resistance training or weight training) makes your body strong and lean. When training for strength, you need muscular strength and muscular endurance. Muscular strength is the maximum amount of force that you can generate by a specific muscle or muscle group. You use this type of strength if you are lifting something very heavy around the house, such as when moving a refrigerator. Muscular endurance, on the other hand, is the ability of your muscles to sustain an activity for a period of time. You employ this type of strength if you are doing an activity that involves physical effort but sustained over a period of time, such as when digging a hole to plant a tree in your yard or shoveling snow in your driveway.

So why do we do strength training exercises? The human body was designed for movement. You have approximately 700 skeletal muscles and this accounts for approximately 23% of a woman's body weight and more than 40% of a man's body weight. At about age 30, your muscle strength declines at a rate of 10 to 15% per decade. Keep your muscle power and get those 700 muscles engaged with our strength program.

What Equipment Do I Need?

Exercise elastic bands (also called resistance or stretch bands or cords): Several manufacturers make exercise elastic bands and they range from easy to hard depending on the color of the bands. For example, Thera-Band has exercise bands with a color range of yellow (easiest) to red, green, blue, or black (hardest). For the exercises described in this book, you are typically going to use 4 feet of elastic band and range from green to blue resistance (based on the Thera-Band resistances).

Dumbbells: Everyone's strength levels vary, of course, and we'll talk later in the chapter about how to gauge how much weight to use for each exercise. For this program, we suggest that women start with 3 to 5 lb dumbbells and men start with 7 to 10 lbs. If you are experienced with strength training, then start with the weights you are accustomed to.

Swiss exercise ball (also called exercise, fitness, or stability balls): The size of these exercise balls vary according to the person's height. Several manufacturers make these balls in different sizes. For example, Thera-Band makes four sizes of balls: 18 inch (45 cm) for a person who is 4'7" to 5'0"; 21 inch (55 cm) for a person who is 5'1" to 5'6"; 26 inch (65 cm) for a person who is 5'2" to 6'1"; 30 inch (75 cm) for a person who is 6'2" to 6'8" in height.

Platform or box: Use a 4 to 6 inch height platform, box, or step.

Exercise gloves (optional): Gloves typically help you get a better grip, especially when using the elastic exercise bands and the dumbbells.

Am I Too Old to Train with Weights?

You're in luck because age is not really an issue. Sarcopenia, or loss of muscle mass is primarily the result of a sedentary lifestyle. With aging we have some physiological declines that lead to muscle loss, but the gains that you can make from strength training are instrumental in keeping you mobile and independent. A study by Maria Fiatarone, MD, at Tufts University in Boston, showed that elderly men and women ages 86 to 96 benefited from weight training to build muscle and improve strength and functional mobility for activities of daily living. In another study, Fiatarone and her colleagues also showed that for frail nursing home men and women residents, ages ranging from 72 to 98, performing high-intensity resistance training was a feasible and effective way of counteracting muscle weakness and physical frailty. Other studies found that resistance training was an effective antidepressant in depressed elders. So no more excuses about being too old to exercise.

What Is Considered Strength Training Exercise?

In strength training (or resistance training), you exercise the muscles of the body to increase strength, power, and muscular endurance through moving a load or weight. Strength training exercises include machines (such as chest press or lat pulldown machine), body weight exercises (such as pull-ups, push-ups, or abdominal curls), free weights (such as barbells or dumbbells), elastic bands, Swiss exercise balls, or water resistance.

How Hard (and Fast) Should I Do Strength Training Exercises?

Your strength training program should be rhythmic, performed at moderate-to-low speed involving full range-of-motion movements that do not interfere with normal breathing. In general, lift for 2 to 3 seconds and lower for at least 2 to 3 seconds. The key is controlled movement with good form and posture. In addition, it's important to remember to breathe! It's pretty common for people to hold their breath while strength training. Instead, concentrate on a breathing pattern of a 2 to 3 second inhale during the lift phase and a 2 to 3 second exhale through the lowering phase or simply count your reps out loud to prevent holding your breath.

How Often Should I Do Strength Training Exercises?

Biceps like Arnold's? Quads like Lance's? Strength training can be an amazing tool for sculpting your body, but keep your expectations reasonable. Too much too fast will only court an injury. Aim for 2 to 3 days per week. Typically, strength workouts can range from 30 to 60 minutes.

You can even increase strength by training for only one day per week. Naturally, this will not yield the same strength results as when training 2 to 3 days per week but it is better than not training at all.

Make sure you take 48 hours between strength workouts to allow your body to recover. Don't forget that rest and recovery from workouts are just as important for good health as doing the exercises. Resistance or strength training causes a mechanical stress to the muscles which results in disruptions or damage to the muscle fibers. This in turn initiates a modification in the muscle proteins. The rest period between exercise sessions allows the muscle fibers to repair and remodel the involved muscle fibers.

How Many Strength Training Exercises Should I Do in Each Workout, and in What Order?

Aim for 8 to 10 separate exercises, which train the major muscle groups (the legs, hips, upper back, shoulder, chest, arms, abdomen, and lower back). Generally, no more than 2 exercises per body area are needed. Make sure you exercise both sides of the body in order to prevent muscle imbalances. Vary the exercises for each body part either every workout or every week. If you are a beginner, start with your arm and other upper body exercises, then do your leg and lower body exercises, and finish with your abs and back. Since you will use your abdominal and back muscles as stabilizers in all your exercises, this will prevent you from overworking them.

In the program we present in Part II, we recommend that you train your largest muscle groups first, where you start with the legs, upper back, chest, shoulders and then work your smaller muscles such as the arms. The exception here is to train your lower back and abdominals last so these muscles do not become fatigued to the point where they are unable to provide stability for your spine. Your abs and lower back are also known as your core muscles; strengthening them will protect against injuries during activities of daily living. Having strong abdominals will allow you to "lock and load" the abdominals during times when you have to lift, push, pull, or carry something heavy.

How Many Sets and Repetitions of Strength Training Exercises Should I Perform?

Rep, set, go! A set is the number of separate exercise bouts that are performed. A repetition (or rep) is the number of times an exercise is performed in succession. You can vary the number of sets and reps you do in order to increase and decrease the intensity of your exercise, as needed. If you are under 50 years of age, aim for sets of 8 to 12 reps with heavier weights; if you are 50 or older, go for 10 to 15 reps with lighter weights.

Most exercise studies suggest that multiple sets are best for optimal strength gains, but 1 set of an exercise is better than none. For the purpose of our program, we recommend you aim for 1 to 3 sets depending on your level of fitness, available time and goals

Between each set, rest for 30 seconds to 3 minutes, depending on your level of fitness, intensity of the exercise, and your goals. If your goal is maximum strength, you should take longer rest periods (for example, 2 to 3 minutes or longer). If your goal is to improve muscle endurance and muscle tone, then shorter rest periods (30 to 60 seconds) may be all you need. The rest periods between sets allow your muscles to recuperate before you challenge them again. The key is to rest long enough so that you use good form in all of your sets. There is no finish line to cross, so take your time and do it right so you don't get injured and you enjoy the workout. For your home program we recommend a 1-minute rest between sets.

How Much Weight Should I Use for Each Strength Training Exercise?

Begin by using your body weight for some exercises (such as pushups, squats, abdominal curls). Then progress to using a weight (such as dumbbells) or elastic resistance with which you can complete at least 10 to 15 reps with good form but no pain. By your last rep, you should feel like you can't physically do another rep; this is known as muscle fatigue. After two weeks of strength training, you should reassess the difficulty of each exercise with your current level of weights (or elastic resistance) and increase to a weight with which you can complete eight reps to the point of fatigue with good form but no pain.

Then, when you've progressed to the point that you are doing 12 to 15 reps without pain, difficulty, or fatigue and while maintaining good form, increase the weights again. Increase the weight by 2.5 to 10%. Or, add 2.5 to 10 pounds for the upper body and 5 to 15 pounds for the lower body. However, if the additional weight causes pain in the joints or aggravates a pre-existing injury, drop down to the lower weight. Remember, this isn't a competition and you're not being paid by how much you lift. Train without pain and train to feel good!

Also, remember that you don't have to keep increasing the amount of weight you use. Stop increasing the weight if:

- you are experiencing pain
- you can't maintain proper form
- a further increase in weight puts your health at risk (for example, if you have a heart condition)
- your doctor specifically advises you that lifting heavy weights puts you at risk (for example, if you have a brain aneurysm or had a brain hemorrhage or heart attack)
- you are satisfied with your strength level, appearance, or how you feel

Are There Things I Should Avoid When Lifting Weights?

Don't try to mimic sports skills with weights, such as swinging a weighted golf club or tennis racket. This practice may lead to injury. Stick to the basic training guidelines we outlined for your safety. Remember to pace your reps, use proper timing of each rep and plan adequate rest between sets. Some athletes lift weights fast, but don't try this at home.

Strength Training Exercises

If you've done any strength training, you'll notice that some very common exercises are missing from this program. For this program, we've deliberately omitted exercises that can potentially create pain or problems in the future. Lunges, for instance, can significantly increase pressure on your knee joint if not done with proper form; deadlifts can exacerbate back and hip pain; and chest flyes may impinge on the shoulder. This doesn't mean that these are bad exercises, only that they are exercises that can affect joints that are most likely to have problems as you get older. If you can work with a physical therapist or personal trainer to be certain that you use proper form and that these exercises do not impact you adversely, by all means feel free to substitute them. Otherwise, it's best to stick with the exercises in this program. Remember, the key is to take things slowly and carefully to avoid injury.

Heel Raises

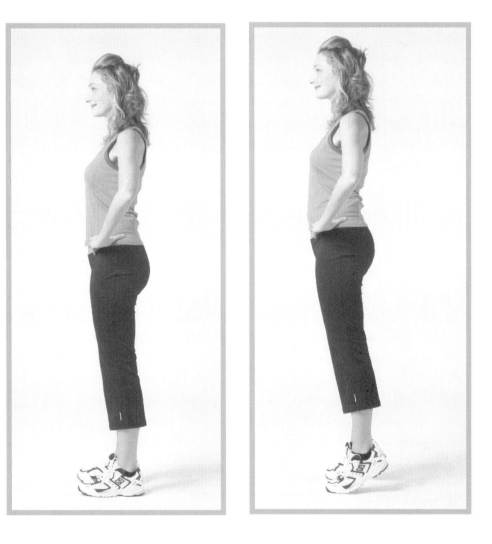

PRECAUTION: **Hang onto something solid if you need to keep your balance.**

62

Purpose: Strengthen the calf muscles and challenge your balance.

Form: Start in a standing position, rise up onto your heels, and lower down slowly.

Frequency: Do 1 to 3 sets of 8 to 15 reps.

Sit-to-Stand Squats

PRECAUTION: Skip this exercise if it causes knee pain.

63

Chapter 5
Your Strength Training and Balance Exercises

Purpose: Strengthen the thigh muscles, directly targeting the quadriceps and indirectly targeting the buttocks and hamstrings.

Form: Start by standing with legs hip width apart. Begin with your arms by your sides. Slowly squat down partially to where your knees are about at a 45-degree bend; at the same time, have your arms come up to the front of your body to chest level to give you balance. Then slowly return to your standing position, feeling your quads, hamstrings and buttocks working. As you squat up and down, slowly keep your knees behind your toes to minimize pressure to your knees.

Frequency: Do 1 to 3 sets of 8 to 15 reps.

Wall Ball Squats

LEGS

64

Purpose: Strengthen the thigh muscles, directly targeting the quadriceps and indirectly targeting the buttocks and hamstrings.

Form: Start by placing a large exercise ball against a wall and then place your back against the ball. Position your feet shoulder width apart and squat down partially to where your thighs remain slightly above the parallel position. Place your hands on your hips and look straight ahead to maintain good posture.

Frequency: Do 1 to 3 sets of 8 to 15 reps.

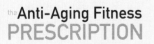

the Anti-Aging Fitness
PRESCRIPTION

Partial Step-Ups

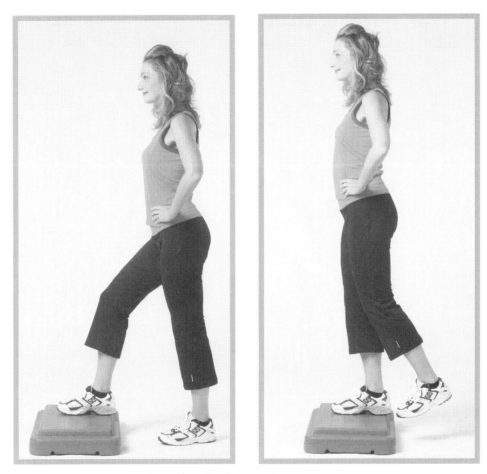

Purpose: Strengthen the thigh muscles.

Form: Start by standing. Place in front of you a box or step that is about 6 inches thick. (You can also create a platform with one or two phone books that are securely taped together to prevent slipping.) Place your right foot on the box and your left foot on the floor. Slowly step up and down with your right leg by keeping your right foot flat, your torso straight and your knees behind your toes as you move up and down. Use a 4 inch height if 6 inches is either too difficult or painful. Repeat on the left leg. Place your hands on your hips.

Frequency: Do 1 to 3 sets of 8 to 15 reps.

PRECAUTION: Skip this exercise if it causes knee or hip pain.

65

Chapter 5
Your Strength Training and Balance Exercises

BACK

66

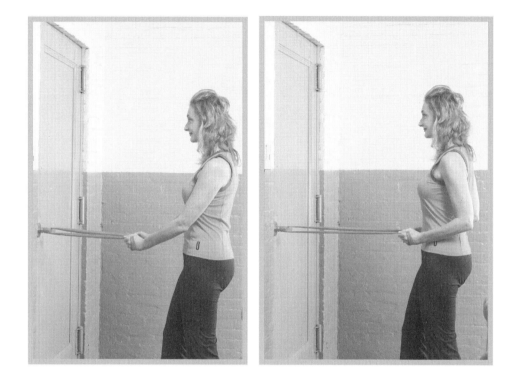

Purpose: Strengthen upper back.

Form: Start by standing with one foot in front of the other with your feet shoulder width apart. Attach an elastic band to a doorknob or solid pole at approximately waist height. With your palms facing inward, pull on the end of the elastic band toward your shoulders in a rowing-type motion.

Frequency: Do 1 to 3 sets of 8 to 15 reps.

Elastic Pull to Hips

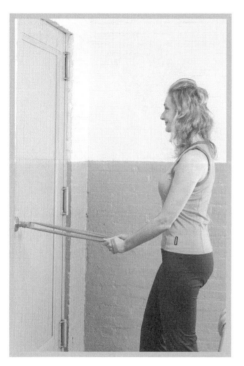 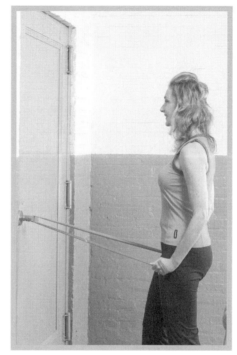

Purpose: Strengthen upper back, lower back, and abdominal muscles.

Form: Start by standing with one foot in front of the other with your feet shoulder width apart. Attach an elastic band to a doorknob or solid pole at approximately waist height. With your palms facing inward, elbows slightly bent, pull on the end of the elastic band toward the sides of your hips.

Frequency: Do 1 to 3 sets of 8 to 15 reps.

PRECAUTION: Avoid shrugging the shoulders upward. Avoid overreaching from the starting position to where your shoulders round forward and pulling your hands too far back to the point where they go past the back of your hips at the ending position.

NOTE: You can also perform this exercise from a seated position.

67

Chapter 5

Your Strength Training and Balance Exercises

Supine Bridging

BACK

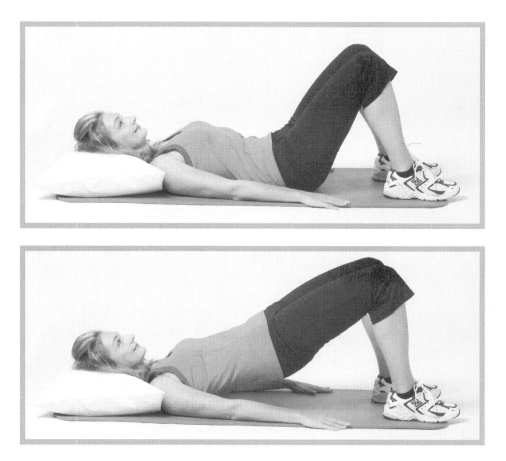

PRECAUTION: Raise your lower back off the floor about the length of your hand to prevent straining your neck and lower back. Skip this exercise if it causes lower back pain.

68

Purpose: Strengthen the muscles in the back of the leg, lower back, and buttocks.

Form: Start by lying on your back, with a pillow or towel under your head, your knees bent and feet shoulder width apart. Raise your hips off the floor about the length of a hand, then slowly lower back down to the floor.

Frequency: Do 1 to 3 sets of 8 to 15 reps.

the Anti-Aging Fitness
PRESCRIPTION

Side Bridging

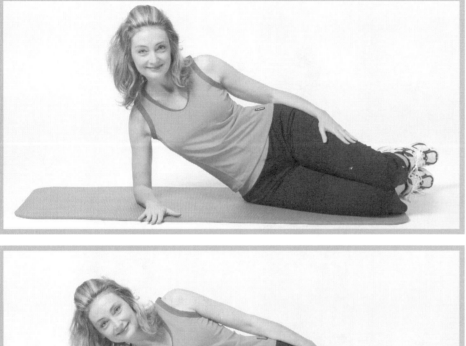

Purpose: Strengthen the muscles in the lower back and abdominals.

Form: Start by lying on your side with your knees bent and supporting yourself on your forearm. Slowly raise your hips up so that your trunk is in a straight position and you are supporting yourself from your forearm and your knees, and hold.

Frequency: Do 1 to 3 sets of a 5- to 15-second hold on each side.

Wingspan Elastic Pulls

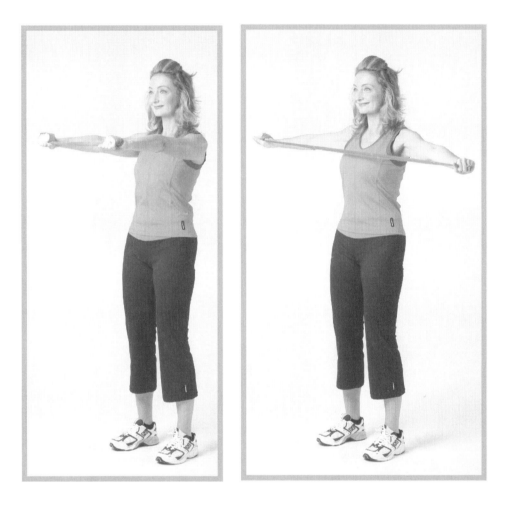

Purpose: Strengthen the shoulder muscles.

Form: Start by standing with your arms straight and raised up to shoulder height in front of you as you hold an elastic band at shoulder width apart. Pull the elastic band apart toward your chest with your palms down and then, slowly return to starting position.

Frequency: Do 1 to 3 sets of 8 to 15 reps.

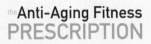

Elastic Outward Rotation

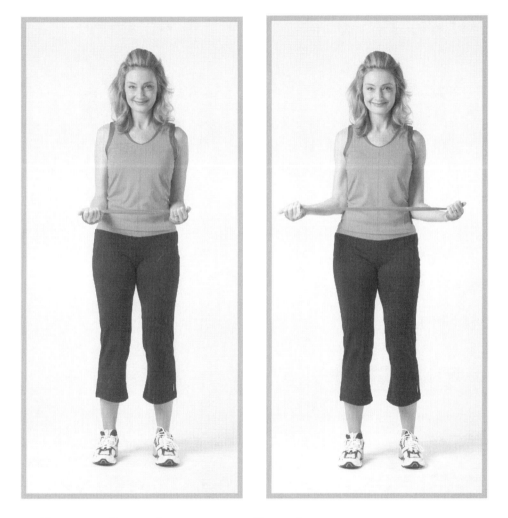

Purpose: Strengthens rotator cuff muscles.

Form: Start in a standing position with your elbows tucked in by your side and bent so that your forearms are parallel to the ground. Grasp the elastic band starting at shoulder width apart with your palms up and thumbs pointing outward, pull the band apart to a comfortable level, and slowly return to the starting position.

Frequency: Do 1 to 3 sets of 8 to 15 reps.

Dumbbell Overhead Press

SHOULDERS AND CHEST

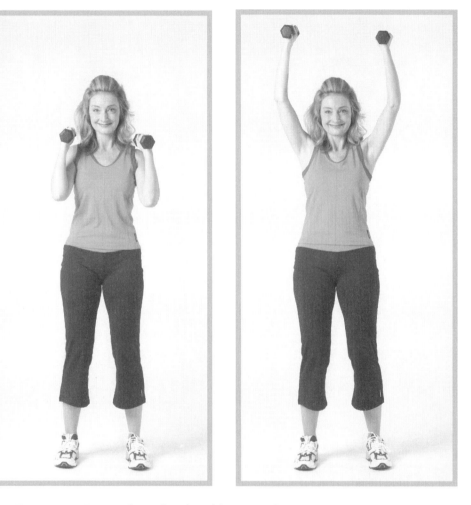

PRECAUTION: **Skip this exercise if it causes shoulder or neck pain. You will often see this exercise done with the palms facing forward, rather than facing each other, but this position causes fewer shoulder impingement problems.**

72

Purpose: Strengthen the shoulder muscles.

Form: Start by standing with your feet shoulder width apart with the dumbbells at shoulder level height and with your palms facing in towards the body. Slowly raise the arms overhead.

Frequency: Do 1 to 3 sets of 8 to 15 reps.

Dumbbell Chest Press

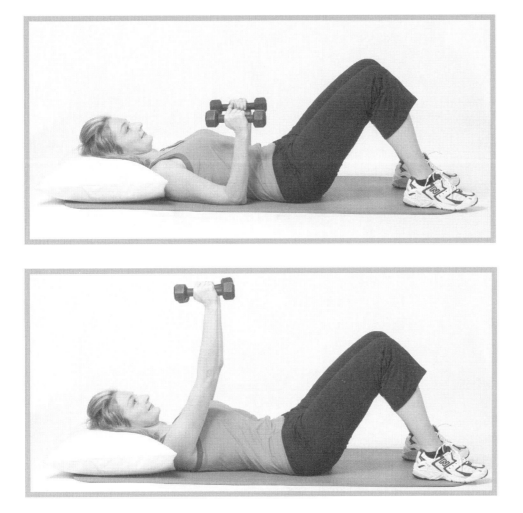

PRECAUTION: **Skip this exercise if it causes shoulder pain. You will often see this exercise done with the palms facing forward, rather than facing each other, but this position causes fewer shoulder impingement problems.**

Purpose: Strengthen the chest and shoulder muscles.

Form: Start by lying on your back with a pillow under your head and your elbows close to your body. Bring dumbbells toward the ceiling with palms facing each other.

Frequency: Do 1 to 3 sets of 8 to 15 reps.

73

Chapter 5

Your Strength Training and Balance Exercises

Modified Pushups

SHOULDERS AND CHEST

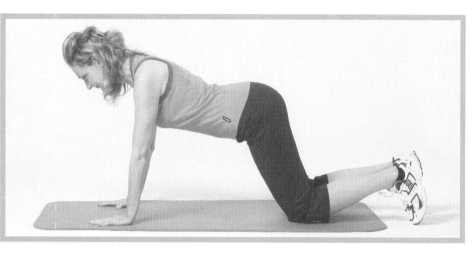

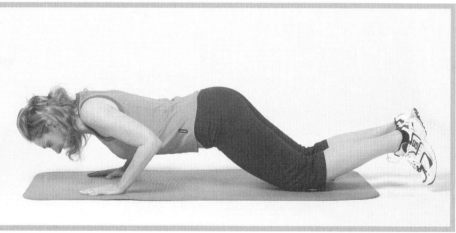

74

Purpose: Strengthen the chest and shoulder muscles, back, and abdominals.

Form: Start by lying face down and place your hands shoulder width apart on the floor. Push your chest off the floor while keeping your knees on the floor.

Frequency: Do 1 to 3 sets of 8 to 15 reps.

Elastic Triceps Pushdown

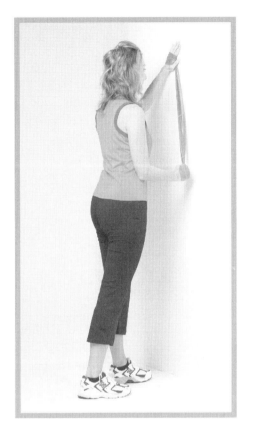

PRECAUTION: **Skip this exercise if it causes shoulder pain to raise your hand to an overhead position.**

75

Chapter 5
Your Strength Training and Balance Exercises

Purpose: Strengthen the muscle on the back of the upper arm.

Form: Stand facing a wall. Wrap the elastic band around your left hand and raise your left hand to a slightly overhead position and place your hand against the wall. Grasp the elastic band with your right hand and bend your elbow so your elbow is by your side and your right hand is at chest height. Now straighten your right elbow so you feel the muscles on the back of your arm working. Repeat with your left arm.

Frequency: Do 1 to 3 sets of 8 to 15 reps.

ARMS

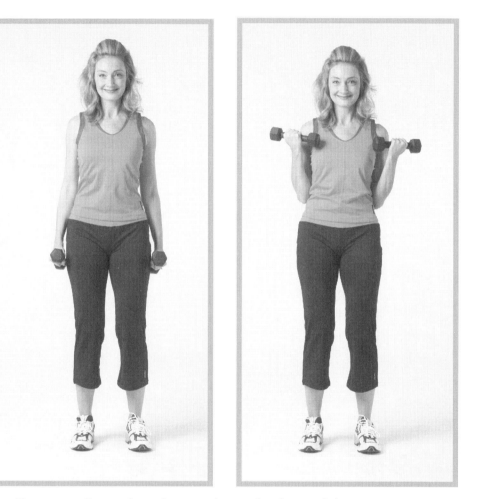

Purpose: Strengthen the muscle on the front of the upper arm.

Form: Start by standing with your feet shoulder width apart and both dumbbells hanging by your hips with your palms facing toward the body. Slowly bend your elbow while slightly rotating the dumbbell outward as you bring the dumbbells towards your shoulders. As you perform the exercise from beginning to end, keep your elbows by your side.

Frequency: Do 1 to 3 sets of 8 to 15 reps.

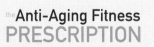

Abdominal Bracing

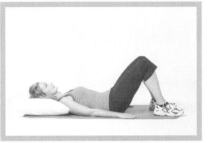
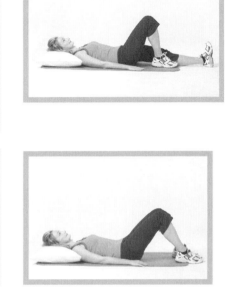

PRECAUTION: Although it may seem like an easy thing to do during the day to work your abs, do not keep the abdominal muscles tightened all the time for prolonged periods during normal day to day tasks. This is not healthy since it interferes with normal relaxed diaphragmatic breathing. However, you should tighten the lower abdominal muscles for physical tasks such as lifting, pushing, pulling, carrying, reaching, as well as for sports activities and for performing the exercises. Do not hold your breath during this exercise.

Chapter 5

Your Strength Training and Balance Exercises

Purpose: Strengthen the abdominal muscles.

Form: Start by lying on your back with a pillow or towel under your head and your knees bent. Take a relaxed breath in and out. As soon as you exhale, tighten your lower abdominal muscles and draw them in towards your spine slightly at the same time you reach the end point of exhaling and then continue to breathe naturally. Do not move your spine or pelvis. Use no more than 30 to 50% effort to tighten your abdominal muscles. Perform the following movements while keeping the lower abdomen tight.

a) Alternate Leg Slides. Start with both knees bent with feet hip width apart. Then, lower one leg to straight position and return to bent knee position. Repeat on the other side.

b) Knees Apart and In. Start with both knees bent with feet hip width apart. Slowly bring knees apart comfortably and then bring knees back together.

Frequency: Do each position for 10 to 30 seconds.

Floor Abdominal Curls

ABDOMINALS

78

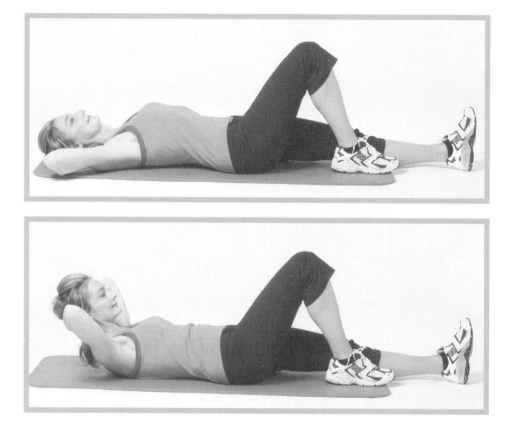

Purpose: Strengthen the abdominal muscles.

Form: Start by lying on your back with one knee bent and one knee straight. Place your hands behind your neck for support and slowly curl up to lift your shoulder blades off the ground slightly. After completing one set, switch leg positions.

Frequency: Do 1 to 3 sets of 8 to 15 reps.

Exercise Ball Abdominal Curls

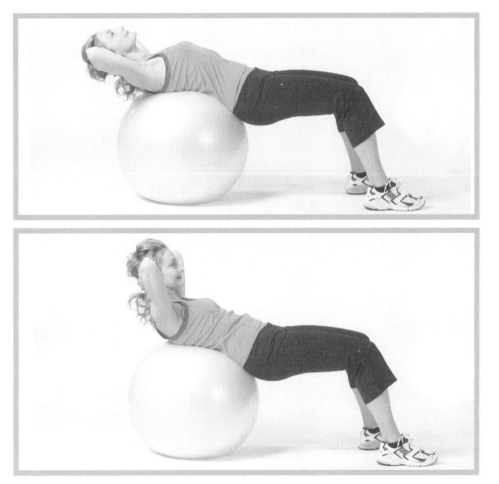

PRECAUTION: **Skip this exercise if you don't have good balance on the ball. Start with the other abdominal exercises and later consider progressing to this more advanced version. When performing this exercise, keep your surrounding area free of clutter and sharp edges in the event you lose your balance. If you have osteoporosis or a back or neck injury, then consult with your healthcare provider or physical therapist before you try this exercise.**

79

Chapter 5

Your Strength Training and Balance Exercises

Purpose: Strengthen the abdominal muscles.

Form: Start by lying down on the exercise ball with your midback against the ball and feet shoulder width apart on the floor. Place your hands behind your neck for support and slowly curl up to lift your shoulder blades off the ball slightly.

Frequency: Do 1 to 3 sets of 8 to 15 reps.

PELVIC FLOOR

NOTE: This exercise, which is for women only, is commonly referred to as Kegels. It is named after the concepts put forth by the late American gynecologist Arnold H. Kegel, MD. He was the pioneer who, over 50 years ago, proposed pelvic floor muscle exercises to prevent and/or treat female urinary incontinence. Today Kegels are also used for overall pelvic floor strengthening after pregnancy and for pelvic floor muscle tone.

80

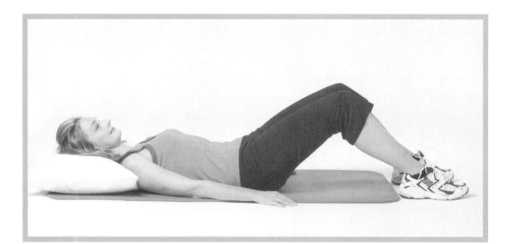

Purpose: Strengthen the pelvic floor muscles.

Form: Start by either sitting or lying down on your back (with a pillow or towel under your head) or side with your knees bent. Keep your legs apart comfortably and your chest relaxed for normal breathing. Now tighten your pelvic floor muscles, and also feel the additional squeeze from the sides as your sphincters (circular muscle fibers formed around your vagina, urethra and anus) tighten and the inside walls move closer together. Breathe naturally during the exercise.

Frequency: Start with 5 to 10 reps for 5 to 10 seconds. Once you have mastered the exercise, physical therapist Elizabeth Noble, who wrote *Essential Exercises for the Childbearing Year,* recommends you perform at least 50 contractions daily.

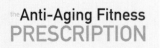

Balance Exercises

As we get older and our bodies heal more slowly, balance becomes more of a concern. Unfortunately, falls are a major concern for people as they get older; among other things, they are the primary reason for many of the hip fractures every year, which can result in lost mobility and reduced independence in daily activities. The balance exercises outlined in this section will help improve your stability and reduce your chance of a fall. See also Day 48 in the Eight-Week-Anti-Aging Fitness Prescription for the How To Prevent A Fall section for more information about preventing falls.

Very Slow Motion Balancing and Walking in Place

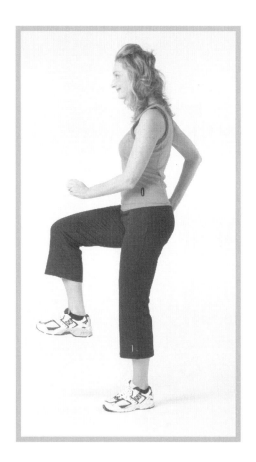

PRECAUTION: **If you are unable to stand and balance on one leg, then skip this exercise and try the modified Dancer's Balance exercise where your toe touches the floor. Next time you are at your physician's office, mention your balance difficulty; your doctor may want you to see a physical therapist for a specific balance training program.**

82

Purpose: Improve overall balance to help prevent falls. Also can help to increase stability/strength of the knees, hips, and lower back.

Form: Start by walking in place very slowly by lifting your knee up to hip level and then repeat on other side. Bring each leg up and down slowly. Hang onto something solid if you need to help keep your balance.

Frequency: Do for 1 to 3 sets of 30 to 60 seconds on each leg.

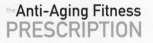

the **Anti-Aging Fitness**
PRESCRIPTION

Dancer's Balance

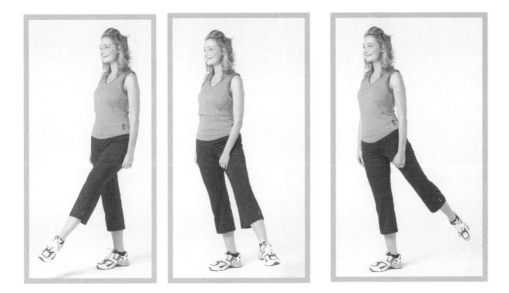

Purpose: Improve overall balance to help prevent falls. Also can help to increase stability/strength of the knees, hips, and lower back. Helps tone your hip and buttocks muscle.

Form: Start by placing your hands on your hips and standing on your right leg. Point your left toes and slowly sweep your left leg forward until it is a few inches off the floor. Be sure to keep your knee straight. Bring your left leg back to center but don't let your left foot touch the floor.

Now point your left toes again and slowly sweep your left leg out to the left side until it is a few inches off the floor. Again, keep your knee straight. Bring your left leg back to center but don't let your left foot touch the floor.

Without stopping, point your left toes and slowly sweep your left leg backwards until it is a few inches off the floor. Again, keep your knee straight. Repeat the same sequence with your right leg. Hang onto something solid if you need to help keep your balance.

Frequency: Take 1 to 2 seconds to perform each position (front, side, and back) and progress to where you perform the exercise for 1 to 3 sets of 30 to 60 seconds total on each leg.

PRECAUTION: If this is too difficult, let your toe touch when you go forward, sideways, and backwards for extra balance.

83

Chapter 5

Your Strength Training and Balance Exercises

Chapter 6

Your Anti-Aging Nutrition Basics

Shoot for Three

Great things come in threes. The Three Stooges, Three Kings, Three Musketeers, Three Dog Night, and the three-point shot in basketball. Keep it simple and think three for anti-aging nutrition. That's three meals, three different colors of fruits and vegetables, and three servings of calcium-rich foods every day. The rationale? In a nutshell, have at *least* three meals a day to fuel your body and keep you on track with healthy food choices, get plenty of disease-fighting phytochemicals and bone-building vitamins with a variety of fruits and vegetables, and maintain your bone density and manage your blood pressure with calcium-rich foods. The nutrition diaries in Part II will make sense of these recommendations and help guide you every day with a suggested menu.

There are many reasons why the quality of our diet wanes with age; our appetite may decline with illnesses, children move out of the house, or perhaps we lose a spouse, limiting our interaction with others at mealtimes so that we eat fewer and less nutritious meals. Eating less and making poor food choices can mean greater incidence of disease, less energy, and generally poor health.

Three Meals a Day

Some people don't like to take the time to prepare meals. Eating is nothing more than a nuisance for them and they end up eating only once or twice a day. They're missing out on an opportunity to get some anti-aging nutrition in their day. Studies show that eating breakfast and having a regular meal rhythm is associated with weight loss and successful weight maintenance.

You'll burn calories just by eating since food requires energy to be digested. This is known as the thermogenic effect of food. Meal skippers lose a little of this calorie-burning effort. They often end up ravenous, and they consume more total calories for the day than if they'd planned ahead and had three meals. If you wait until you're starving, it's not likely that you'll make healthy food choices including fruits and vegetables. Instead, you may reach for high-calorie fast food or something from the vending machine that has very little nutritional value. A little planning for your three meals a day will allow you to add fruits and vegetables and calcium-rich foods with ease.

Three Different Colored Fruits and Vegetables Every Day

Through years of counseling clients, we've met dozens of people who report that they love fruits and vegetables. But when we look at their seven-day food record, we routinely find that they have only eaten one to two servings of fruits or vegetables during the *entire week*. They're shocked when we point out the dismal intake of produce. Our favorite was a woman who professed her love of spinach, going on about it for minutes, until we finally asked her how often she eats it. She couldn't even recall the last time she ate spinach.

Fruits and vegetables contain phytochemicals, non-nutritive plant chemicals that contain disease-preventive compounds. Nine hundred phytochemicals have been identified and more are being discovered through current research. By including diverse vegetables and fruits in your diet you can protect yourself against certain types of cancer, heart disease, diabetes, premature aging, vision loss, and dementia. Choose three different colored fruits and three different colored vegetables to have every day. We'll guide you in adding fruits and vegetables to your diet in Part II, where you'll also find the "Color Your World" table, which lists different colored fruits and their health benefits.

A good plan is to have two servings of fruit at breakfast and one fruit for a snack, one serving of vegetable at lunch and two servings of vegetables at dinner. You can always have more, but if you're starting from ground zero, take it gradually and work up to six servings a day. It sounds like a lot of rabbit food, but it's pretty easy to do. Keep in mind that a serving does not necessarily mean a heaping plateful of vegetables. The American Cancer Society gives these guidelines, which are easy to remember and accepted by the healthcare community as being good for general health (not just to prevent cancer or help cancer patients), for portions of fruits and vegetables:

- One vegetable serving: 1 cup raw or ½ cup cooked
- One fruit serving: 1 medium whole fruit, 1 cup berries or cut fruit, ¼ cup dried fruit, ½ cup water- or juice-packed canned fruit

In addition to the nutrients you get from all of these fruits and vegetables, you'll find that all this low-calorie, high-fiber food will fill you up, so there won't be much room left for junk food. And, as an added bonus, the fruits and vegetables will boost your water intake. When you put them at the forefront of your meal planning, you'll simply find that you eat them. And that's the goal right there.

A Word about Juices

Many people will eye this list of fruits and vegetables and proclaim, well, I'm going to get a juicer, juice all of my fruits and vegetables, and get them in one fell swoop. While I can't deny that 100% fruit and vegetable juices contain phytochemicals, they are not recommended to fulfill these servings on a daily basis. You'll miss out on the valuable fiber in the fruit or vegetable by choosing juice. Also, liquids don't satisfy and fill you

up like eating the whole fruit or vegetable, and a serving is quite small, just 4 to 6 ounces depending on the juice. Fruit juices can raise your blood sugar level quickly and dramatically. I would not recommended fruit juice for people with diabetes. Juice is OK for occasional use, but not to routinely fulfill your three-a-day requirement.

Totally Radical

Free radicals can damage our DNA and cell membrane, ultimately leading to disease. Antioxidants can block the pathway of free radicals, limiting the harm they do to our body. ORAC, short for Oxygen Radical Absorbance Capacity, measures the ability of food and other substances to subdue free radicals in the test tube. A diet rich in high-ORAC activity foods can raise the antioxidant power of human blood. In animal studies, these foods can prevent long-term memory problems and enhance

Top Antioxidant Foods

FRUITS	ORAC	VEGETABLES	ORAC
Prunes	5,770	Kale	1,770
Raisins	2,830	Spinach	1,260
Blueberries	2,400	Brussel sprouts	980
Blackberries	2,036	Alfalfa sprouts	930
Strawberries	1,540	Broccoli florets	890
Raspberries	1,220	Beets	840
Plums	949	Red bell pepper	710
Oranges	750	Onion	450
Grapes, red	739	Corn	400
Cherries	670	Eggplant	390

* ORAC (Oxygen Radical Absorbance Capacity) – units per 100 grams (about 3.5 ounces)

Vitamin K is OK

Your production of bone matrix is dependent on vitamin K. You can do your bones a favor by exploring ways to get adequate vitamin K in your daily food intake. The "green group" in the *Color Your World* chart lists foods high in vitamin K and other foods rich in K include cauliflower, chick peas, dairy products, eggs, seeds and olive and canola oil.

Few food/drug interactions are as well-known, and feared, as the interaction between vitamin K and blood thinning medications. For the record, these medications don't actually thin the blood, they work as anticoagulants and they help prevent new blood clots from forming. Most of our clients who take anti-coagulants are fearful of eating any green vegetables. But you needn't worry! Talk to your doctor about how to get a steady intake of vitamin K in your diet. Also, ask your doctor about INR testing. "The physician should regulate the patient's use of anti-coagulants with INR (the International Normalized Ratio). It's essential that monitoring be done," reports Joseph R. Robinson, MD, a cardiologist at The Washington Hospital Center in Washington, DC, and a proponent of a high vegetable intake for all of his patients.

Although vitamin K supplements shouldn't be taken with this medication, you may be able to tolerate a *constant* amount of vitamin K from foods in your daily intake. For those taking anti-coagulant medication, consistency with your vitamin K intake is important, but physician INR management is absolutely essential.

Foods and supplements to completely avoid while taking an anticoagulant include green and herbal tea, fish oil supplements, soybeans and soybean oil, alcohol, caffeine and fried or boiled onions. Every single supplement you take needs to be approved by your doctor, so always have a list ready to share with your doctor of every pill that passes your lips.

learning ability, maintain the ability of brain cells, and protect capillaries from oxygen damage.

Three Calcium-Rich Foods Per Day

Less than half of Americans get enough calcium every day. And our need for calcium increases as we get older. Most of us know by now that calcium is crucial to building and maintaining bone density and avoiding osteoporosis, which affects 25 million Americans. But did you know that calcium is also a key ingredient to battling high blood pressure? Over one third of Americans age 45 and older have high blood pressure, which puts us at risk for stroke, heart disease and congestive heart failure. Adequate calcium, along with potassium, magnesium, protein, and fiber, is critical for blood pressure management. Therefore, we recommend that you get at least three calcium-rich foods a day.

Small studies by Michael P. Zemel, PhD, a professor of nutrition at the University of Tennessee, suggest that three servings a day of low fat dairy foods such as milk, yogurt and cheese could give a boost to weight loss and weight management. The calcium in dairy appears to shift energy use from storage to oxidation. But are dairy foods a "magic pill" for weight loss? Even the researchers agree that if you don't restrict calories, there is no weight loss associated with increased dairy intake. What if you're overweight and you already consume 800

mg/day of calcium from dairy sources? Unfortunately, you won't lose weight by increasing your dairy consumption.

Most of us think of dairy foods when we think of calcium, and they are certainly a primary source. But they are not the only one. Many foods today are supplemented with calcium, including many breakfast cereals and juices. Some calcium-fortified drinks, however, may not measure up as well to dairy to fulfill this calcium requirement. For example, soy milk or rice milk fortified with calcium may not have enough calcium suspended in the liquid to allow for absorption.

"The calcium that you'll find added to many soy beverages will have settled to the bottom of the container," said Robert P. Heaney, MD, FACP, FACN, of the Osteoporosis Research Center at Creighton University, Omaha. "Hand shaking wasn't enough; we found that really vigorous shaking, such as with a hardware store paint shaker, would have been needed to suspend the calcium in these beverages so you can put them in the glass and drink them." Now, before you decide to forego any calcium-fortified drinks, let's look at the whole story. Heaney found that the calcium in Tropicana brand calcium-fortified orange juice is suspended well in the liquid and is available for absorption.

In addition, dark green and cruciferous vegetables, such as collard greens and turnip greens, are rich in calcium. "The calcium in cruciferous vegetables is well absorbed," Heaney states. And you don't need us to tell you what nutritional powerhouses these foods are. You'll get your phytochemicals, vitamin K, and calcium to boot!

Ultimately, your goal should be to get 1200 mg calcium per day from the foods you eat or drink. You can even slip in this amount of calcium in two servings of superfoods. See the table Cool Calcium Choices on page 163 for the calcium content of the anti-aging recipes and other foods. In order for your body to utilize calcium, you also need enough vitamin D.

More D Please!

Vitamin D is a fat-soluble vitamin found in food but your body can also synthesize it from exposure to sunlight. It acts as a hormone by sending a message to your intestines to absorb calcium and phosphorus. Without enough D, bones become brittle, thin, and misshapen. Vitamin D deficiency can be characterized by muscle pain, muscle weakness, and bone pain (symptoms which can prompt a *take it easy* from your physician, and we don't need another reason to stop exercising!). Chronic fatigue syndrome and

fibromyalgia have similar symptoms, and people are often misdiagnosed with these diseases when in fact they may have a vitamin D deficiency. Adequate vitamin D is helpful for some conditions including:

- Mood health: prevents seasonal affective disorder, premenstrual tension, sleeping disorders and improves overall sense of well-being
- Bone health: prevents osteoporosis, osteomalacia, and rickets
- Cellular health: prevents breast, colon, and prostate cancers
- Organ health: prevents heart disease, stroke
- Autoimmune health: prevents multiple sclerosis, type 1 diabetes mellitus, and rheumatoid arthritis

The National Institutes of Health Office of Dietary Supplements (part of the Institute of Medicine of the National Academy of Sciences) set these adequate intake levels for vitamin D. The unit of measure for vitamin D is in International Units, which is how you'll see them listed on a nutrition facts label.

Intake Recommendations

Age (Years)	Men	Women
0-50	200 IU	200 IU
51-70	400 IU	400 IU
71+	600 IU	600 IU
Breastfeeding/Pregnancy		200 IU

HIGH D FOODS

The list of foods rich in vitamin D is short, so it's very difficult to get all the vitamin D you need through foods alone. We'll tell you how to complement your diet with safe sun exposure and supplements, but you may also want to choose a few vitamin D rich foods to include in your eating plan. Many ready-to-eat breakfast cereals are fortified with vitamin D; only one example is listed, but check the label of your favorite cereal.

HOW DO I GET SAFE SUN EXPOSURE?

The National Institutes of Health note that exposure to sunlight provides most humans with their vitamin D requirement. But with all the buzz about the risks of skin cancer, aging skin, and eye damage, you'll want to be very careful about how much sun you get. Michael Holick, PhD, MD, a researcher at Boston University School of Medicine and author of *The UV Advantage,* recommends that you estimate how long it will take you to

get a mild sunburn (for light-skinned people this is when your skin gets pink, and for darker skinned people this is when you skin starts to get darker or reddened). Then, two to three times a week, expose your face, hands, and arms (or arms and legs) for only 20 to 25 percent of that time.

If you are concerned about wrinkling on your face and neck caused by overexposure to the sun, then use a wide-brimmed hat and sunscreen on your face and expose other body parts instead. For example, if it would take thirty minutes for your skin to get pink, darker or reddened in the sunshine, then spend six to eight minutes in the sun before putting on SPF 15 sunscreen. The time it takes for your skin to show this change in the sun is called a minimal erythemal dose (MED). Do this two to three times a week. Holick cautions against sun overexposure in order to prevent skin cancer and skin damage and recommends that after an individual's safe exposure limit that they use sun block

Foods High in Vitamin D

Food	Vitamin D
Salmon, cooked, 3.5 ounces	360 IU
Mackerel, cooked, 3.5 ounces	345 IU
Sardines, canned in oil, drained, 1.75 ounces	250 IU
Chunk Light Tuna, canned in oil, 3 ounces	198 IU
Milk, fat-free and 1%, 1 cup	98 IU
Tropicana Pure Premium Orange Juice Calcium + Vitamin D, 1 cup	98 IU
Total Whole Grain Cereal, ¾ cup or Cheerios, 1 cup	40 IU
Egg, 1 whole (vitamin D is in the yolk)	20 IU

and protective clothing, such as light-colored, tightly woven, long-sleeved shirts and pants.

Always adjust your calculations depending on the situation. For example, if you are at the beach at ten in the morning or four in the afternoon, the sun is less strong, so you can spend longer in the sun without protection. If you estimate that at that time, based on your experience, it would take an hour for you to get one MED, then you can spend about fifteen minutes in the sun without any sunscreen on. Please note that you shouldn't ever try to get a mild sunburn, but estimate how long it would take your skin to turn pink, darker or reddened and then make your

Don't Pass the Salt, Please

There's no room in your anti-aging plan for table salt. Excess sodium in your day is associated with high blood pressure, which can then contribute to hypertension, stroke, heart disease, and kidney disease. Many recipes call for salt, and let's face it, many of us like to sprinkle a little on our food. We're looking for flavor, and you can find it right here with this easy-to-prepare seasoning mixture. Try this seasoning for all of your recipes that call for salt (experiment with portions for the best flavor) and try a sprinkle on your food. Say goodbye to table salt forever.

No-Salt Seasoning

1 tablespoon garlic powder
2 teaspoons sage
2 teaspoons dried basil
2 teaspoons onion powder
2 teaspoons parsley
2 teaspoons thyme
2 teaspoons marjoram
2 teaspoons ground black pepper
1 teaspoon ground red pepper or cayenne pepper (optional)

1 Mix all ingredients well and use a clean, dry spice container with large holes to dispense. For a milder flavor, leave out the cayenne pepper.

calculations of safe sun time accordingly. Also, keep in mind that certain conditions, such as reflections from water, sand, snow, or even grass, or being at higher elevations, can increase your exposure. You can also get sun exposure in the shade or on cloudy days.

Before you go out in the sun, check with your physician if you have a medical condition or take medications that make your skin sensitive to the sun. We also highly recommend that you get periodic checkups from a dermatologist, especially if you spend a lot of time outdoors. Susan Harris, DSc, of the June Mayer Human Nutrition Research Center on Aging at Tufts University, recommends that dark-skinned people in particular consider increasing their vitamin D intake during the short days of winter. See the High D list on page 90 for food sources. In addition, the following groups of people are encouraged to consider vitamin D supplements:

- Adults age 50 to 70, consider taking 400 IU.
- Adults age 71 and older, consider taking 600 IU.
- People with darker skin tone including African Americans and other populations with dark pigmented skin (see Intake Recommendations based on age).
- For infants who are exclusively breastfed and are not exposed to sunlight, 200 IU supplementation is recommended continuing through breastfeeding stage.
- Persons with fat malabsorption, pan-

creatic enzyme deficiency, Crohn's disease, cystic fibrosis, celiac sprue, or surgical removal of part of the stomach or intestines.

Anti-Aging Supplements

Now that you have a guideline for getting most of the nutrients you need from food, it's time to explore the world of supplements. If you looked up "supplements" online, you'd come up with so many hits that it would literally take you months to read everything that comes up. And, unfortunately, the promises of youth and vigor that come along with supplements are usually empty. So with a few exceptions, most notably vitamin D, the evidence for supplementing with every vitamin or mineral under the sun isn't too strong.

So do you need supplements? Healthy people can usually get everything they need from a well-rounded diet. Supplements, including not only vitamins and minerals but also herbals, botanicals, amino acids, enzymes, animal extracts, and other substances, are not intended to make up for a poor diet or lifestyle. Some are well understood, but others need further study.

Don't ever substitute supplements for medications without your physician's approval. Ingesting high levels or mega-doses of vitamins, minerals, protein or other supplements, including herbs, can have serious consequences. Potential side effects with any supplement could include skin rash or hives,

The Claim, The Verdict

Antioxidant Supplement (typically includes any combination of vitamin A, C, B6, B12, E, beta-carotene, folate, selenium)	
THE CLAIM: Benefits for cardiovascular, eye, immune and cognitive health.	THE VERDICT: Large, randomized controlled trials do not support the use of antioxidant supplements for well-nourished older adults. There are possible adverse effects. Research supports that antioxidants should come from fruits and vegetables, not supplements.
Vitamin A	
THE CLAIM: Treatment of xerophthalmia (leads to blindness) and retinitis pigmentosa (impaired night vision and peripheral vision), cancer prevention and boosts immune system.	THE VERDICT: Clinical trials show the anti-oxidant and cancer prevention benefits are unclear. Increased risk of lung cancer for smokers and alcohol users.
Vitamin C	
THE CLAIM: Treatment of asthma, cancer, diabetes, prevention of cataracts, stroke, and heart disease. Prevention and treatment of the common cold and respiratory infections.	THE VERDICT: Studies show no significant benefits for any of these diseases or infections. People living in extreme circumstances such as sub-arctic exercisers, skiers, and marathon runners do realize a 50% reduction in risk of developing the common cold.
Vitamin B6	
THE CLAIM: Prevention and treatment of neuritis, anemia, seizures, asthma, cardio-vascular disease, carpal tunnel syndrome, depression and kidney stones. Improve immune function and prevent stroke reoccurrence.	THE VERDICT: Research supports use of B6 supplement for preventing and treating pyridoxine deficiency and neuritis due to insufficient dietary intake, certain disease states or deficiency induced by drugs, with your doctor's guidance. The evidence is incon-clusive for all other claims.
Vitamin B12	
THE CLAIM: Treatment of pernicious and megaloblastic anemia, Alzheimer's disease, angioplasty (decrease in the rate of restenosis), breast cancer, cardiovascular disease, fatigue, high cholesterol, sleep disorders, lung cancer, stroke reoccurrence, and shaky-leg syndrome.	THE VERDICT: Proven usefulness for pernicious and megaloblastic anemia, with your doctor's guidance. Well-designed clinical trials are needed to validate the use of B12 for all other claims.

The Claim, The Verdict (continued)

Vitamin D	
THE CLAIM: Prevention of rickets in children, osteomalacia in adults, hypertension, some cancers, and autoimmune diseases.	**THE VERDICT:** Supplementation is useful for those at risk for vitamin D deficiency including dark-skinned people, the elderly, exclusively breast-fed infants, people who cover all exposed skin or use sunscreen whenever out-side, and people who have fat malabsorption syndromes (e.g., cystic fibrosis) or inflamma-tory bowel disease (e.g., Crohn's disease).
Vitamin E	
THE CLAIM: Prevention of heart disease, numerous skin diseases, stroke, seizures, res-piratory infection, prostate cancer, PMS, Parkinson's disease, high cholesterol, kidney disease, diabetes, cataracts and other eye diseases, many cancers and anemia.	**THE VERDICT:** Further research is needed to substantiate these many claims. Safety concern of possible increased risk of bleeding particularly you're taking anti-coagulant medication.
Beta-carotene	
THE CLAIM: Prevention of stroke, post-operative tissue injury, cardiovascular disease, cancer, angioplasty, Alzheimer's disease, abdominal aortic aneurysm, sunburn, osteoarthritis, macular degeneration, cataracts, and chronic obstructive pulmonary disease. Treatment of H pylori bacterial infection and erythropoietic protoporphyria.	**THE VERDICT:** Useful for the rare, genetic skin disease, erythropoietic protoporphyria. Addi-tional evidence is needed before conclusions can be drawn with regards to all other claims.
Folate	
THE CLAIM: Prevention or treatment of preg-nancy complications, methotrexate toxicity, Alzheimer's disease, chronic fatigue syndrome, cancer, depression, vascular disease / hyperho-mocysteinemia, vitiligo, and stroke.	**THE VERDICT:** Useful for prevention of pregnancy complications and for people using low-dose, long-term methotrexate for rheumatoid arthritis or psoriasis. Once again, get your doctor's approval. Well-designed clinical trials needed to validate the usefulness of folate for all other conditions.

The Claim, The Verdict (continued)

Selenium

THE CLAIM: Improve mood and provide health benefit for inflammatory or infectious diseases such as rheumatoid arthritis or human immunodeficiency virus/acquired immunodeficiency syndrome, and those who are at high risk for cancers, particularly prostate cancer.

THE VERDICT: Selenium is useful for all of these conditions but you can meet your recommended intake from food alone. If you are a candidate for this supplement, talk to your doctor about taking a multivitamin with 20 to 55 mcg selenium.

Coenzyme Q 10

THE CLAIM: Extend the lifespan with prevention of double-strand DNA breakage. DNA breakage causes a variety of diseases.

THE VERDICT: More research is needed to prove cancer preventive properties. Rat studies show that small dosages can be beneficial for prevention of DNA breakage.

Dehydroepiandrosterone(DHEA)

THE CLAIM: Suggested to slow aging, improve cognition, improve muscle and bone strength, protect against many diseases, prevent cardiovascular disease, and improve immunity.

THE VERDICT: Studies show no benefit and possible liver damage even with short-term use.

Testosterone

THE CLAIM: Supplementation with testosterone is thought to be linked to improved energy level and sex drive, improved muscle strength, and reduced incidence of osteoporosis.

THE VERDICT: No evidence to back up this claim. Possible liver damage.

Melatonin

THE CLAIM: Prevention or treatment of insomnia, jet lag, aging, and cancer. Suggested to improve sex drive.

THE VERDICT: Studies show a benefit for insomnia in the elderly, jet lag, delayed sleep phase syndrome, and sleep enhancement in healthy people. Dosage is very important for these uses, so get guidance from your physician. Studies have been small and short-term and long-term effects are not known.

Human Growth Hormone (HGH)

THE CLAIM: Promises to build muscle, renew energy, increase bone density, and improve mood.

THE VERDICT: Study participants gained muscle mass but no added strength. Unclear benefit for bone density and mood. Side effects include swelling in your arms and legs, headaches, bloating, muscle pain, diabetes, and high blood pressure.

nausea or vomiting, diarrhea or constipation, headaches, dizziness or lightheadedness, breathing difficulties, difficulty sleeping, heart racing or blurry vision. So, if you are going to take over-the-counter supplements, especially in combination with medications or before medical procedures, always consult with your physician regarding possible adverse interactions.

Be wary of these common myths about supplements:

It Can't Hurt Me and It Might Help Me. Not so fast. Some ingredients can be toxic in large amounts (and the recommended dosage sometimes qualifies as a large amount), when taken for a long enough time or in combination with other medications or supplements in your diet.

But I Just Heard about It on the News. The media often reports the findings of single studies. Find out the source of the study, look for long-term studies to establish guidance of dosage and expected health effects, and ask your doctor before you take anything.

It's *Natural*, So Of Course It's Safe! Don't be fooled by the claim "natural." It doesn't mean anything. Supplements are not subject to the strict regulation and testing by the FDA that medications and food receive, and they absolutely can hurt you.

That said, supplements aren't always bad. Your physician or dietitian may recommend temporary or long-term supplement use to ensure that you get the proper nutrients if you have a restricted diet or a specific condition known to be helped by specific nutrients. You may need dietary supplements if you have osteoporosis or if you are on a restricted or low-calorie plan such as a post gastric surgery diet. If you have food allergies, or are traveling to remote wilderness locations where there is limited food available, you may need to round out your intake with a supplement. You may also need some help if you are a vegetarian, a dark-skinned or elderly person living in a northern latitude, or an elite athlete. The bottom line is you should first work on improving your diet with proper foods and only consider supplements when they're prescribed for special circumstances.

Many available supplements and hormones promise to manage diseases associated with aging or halt the aging process altogether. Antioxidants are particularly popular, and we'll examine an antioxidant combination as well as the individual vitamins and minerals. The table on pages XX lists some of the trendier *fountain of youth* pills and potions and sets the record straight.

Putting Your Eating Plan Together

Can you recall with absolute accuracy every morsel you put in your mouths? Most people don't even come close. In fact, the vast majority of us underestimate how much we eat. But how can we enjoy our food if we don't remember eating it? And how can we possibly expect to drop any weight if we really don't know how many calories are going in? A little planning goes a long way to help you manage all of the challenges that come along (eating out, food at work, celebrations) and still keep a healthy weight. Your nutrition diaries provide space to log your foods and many other tips to help you plan your intake. The Eight-Week Anti-Aging Fitness Prescription also guides you in adding different-colored fruits and vegetables, calcium-rich, and vitamin-D-rich foods to your diet.

The National Weight Control Registry has identified thousands of people who have lost weight and kept it off. They found that people who consistently follow an eating plan for each meal and snack showed a much greater likelihood of maintaining their weight loss. You might be thinking, now what's so special about that . . . of course consistency will lead to weight maintenance. But it's actually very telling. Many people who follow an eating plan (particularly fad diet fanatics) relax their boundaries on the weekends or for vacations, and it's really hard to jump back onto your food plan if you have lots of days of overeating. The calories can add up quickly, and it's difficult to continue to lose weight or maintain any weight loss with two completely free eating days per week. We give you a little planned indulgence (see Nutrition Diary Days 4 and 5 for treat guidelines) and this can go a long way to keeping you on track and feeling good about your plan, but too many calories on a regular basis will plateau your weight loss efforts, or worse yet, cause you to gain weight.

....

Tales From the Table:
Map Out Your Meals

Ali, a 36-year-old single woman, complains that she just can't get it together to lose the last 30 pounds. At an all-time high of 188 pounds in college, the 5'2" auburn-haired accountant has been successful at shedding and keeping off 38 pounds for the past ten years. The scale is stuck at 150 pounds, and no amount of exercise seems to make a difference. A consistent exerciser, Ali sweats through a grueling weight workout twice a week for 45 minutes, and cross trains at a moderate or high intensity for at least four cardio workouts a week.

Ali reports, "I eat thawed frozen blueberries, yogurt, and a few nuts for breakfast, I usually get a big salad with lots of grilled vegetables, roasted chicken and a wheat roll for lunch, but by the time I walk in the door at 6:00 p.m. I can't muster the energy to make anything for dinner. I collapse on the couch, watch television and munch on chips and salsa or cookies until they're coming out of my ears. Maybe twice a week I go out and have a healthy dinner with friends. I have the opposite problem that most people have, if I eat out I do fine but if I don't have a meal planned, look out. Weekends can be an all-day calorie fest. I would like to lose 30 pounds and I just can't seem to get the weight loss started."

Ali was exasperated, and finally went to see a Registered Dietitian. She asked Ali to keep a food journal to help her pinpoint what motivates her overeating and to find opportunities for improvement in her existing eating habits. Ali and her dietitian found that her overeating wasn't prompted by emotions or stress, but rather she simply didn't plan well enough for all of her meals. The dietitian recommended making two family-size dinners a week to carry her through her trouble times, weekday dinners and weekends, and to have an emergency supply of healthy frozen meals such as rice bowls with vegetables and lower fat entrees. They worked together to find easy recipes that she could make using many of the same ingredients, and they decided on recipes for a healthy pizza, lasagna, and chili. Ali made these and was shocked at how easy it was to throw together a meal. She didn't like to cook, but now she was saving money and making healthy meals with very little effort.

In two months, Ali was successful at dropping 8 pounds. She had two or three overeating episodes that reflected her old habits, but they were only a result of poor planning. She was amazed to find how easy it was to eat healthfully and be freed from her bingeing ways while reaching her goal of losing weight.

....

Chapter 7

Your Anti-Aging Recipes

A satisfying meal for one or for a whole family can be prepared in minutes. These dishes are designed to meet your goal of getting a variety of different colored fruits and vegetables and adequate calcium. Although you'll find fresh ingredients, you can substitute frozen or canned varieties of fruits and vegetables. If you decide to use convenience items, choose "no salt added" canned vegetables, plain frozen vegetables (without sauce packets), and canned fruit packed in juice or water.

These portions will look enormous since they contain mostly low calorie density foods that pack a lot of water. Don't hesitate to make your serving size smaller if the amount of food seems overwhelming.

In addition to the breakfast, lunch, and dinner recipes, we've included a few spreads to replace sugary dessert toppings, cream cheese, or butter. Smear them on whole wheat toast, a granola bagel, an oat bran English muffin, or even a whole wheat soft tortilla for a quick, healthy breakfast or snack. The ricotta cheese spread sounds kind of, shall we say, unique. Give it a try, you'll be surprised how good it tastes and how versatile it can be in your meal plan. The sour cream spread is sweet enough to top a bowl of berries. Be sure to store the spreads in the refrigerator and use them within about 5 to 6 days after mixing.

For microwave cooking instructions, use full power or "high" unless otherwise noted.

Many recipes call for "no-salt seasoning." See page 91 for the recipe for no-salt seasoning.

Sweet Cottage Cheese Bowl

Serves 1

Ingredients

¾ cup 1% cottage cheese
½ cup low fat fruit-flavored yogurt
½ papaya or 60 calories of your favorite fruit
2 tablespoons low fat granola or Grape Nuts cereal

Directions

1 Mix all ingredients together in a bowl.

Nutrition Facts

Per Serving: 356 calories, 29 g protein, 55 g carbohydrate, 4 g fat, 2 g saturated fat, 841 mg sodium, 12 mg cholesterol, 4 g fiber, 334 mg calcium

Yogurt Bowl

Serves 1

Ingredients

1 cup low fat plain yogurt

½ cup high fiber cereal (with at least 3 grams fiber), 90 calories worth such as Kellogg's Raisin Bran, Kashi Go Lean, or Barbara's Bakery Organic Grainshop Cereal

1 serving fruit, 60 calories worth such as 1 small whole piece fruit, 1 cup chopped fruit, or 2 tablespoons dried fruit

2 tablespoons chopped nuts

Directions

1 In a large bowl, pour in yogurt and add cereal, fruit, and nuts over the top.

Nutrition Facts

Per Serving: 413 calories, 20 g protein, 62 g carbohydrate, 14 g fat, 3 g saturated fat, 243 mg sodium, 15 mg cholesterol, 12 g fiber, 466 mg calcium

Breakfast

Chapter 7

Your Anti-Aging Recipes

Fruit and Cheese Foldover

Serves 1

Ingredients

One 8" whole wheat soft tortilla
4 tablespoons cheddar cheese, shredded
1 thinly sliced pear
A sprinkle of ground cinnamon

Directions

1 Lay out the tortilla and top with the shredded cheese and thinly sliced pear.

2 Sprinkle with a shake of cinnamon if desired and heat in the microwave for 40 to 50 seconds.

3 Roll up or fold to eat.

Nutrition Facts

Per Serving: 271 calories, 7 g protein, 45 g carbohydrate, 8 g fat, 3 g saturated fat, 352 mg sodium, 15 mg cholesterol, 7 g fiber, 246 mg calcium

Fluffy Orange Pancakes

Serves 4 (Makes 20 small pancakes)

Ingredients

1 tablespoon trans-free margarine
1 cup low fat ricotta cheese
2 eggs
2 tablespoons brown sugar
Zest of ½ fresh orange peel (if desired)
½ teaspoon pure vanilla extract
¼ teaspoon ground cinnamon
¼ cup plus 1 tablespoon whole wheat flour
Butter-flavored cooking spray
8 tablespoons light maple syrup

Directions

1. In a bowl, mix together the margarine, ricotta cheese, and eggs. Add brown sugar, zest of fresh orange peel, pure vanilla extract, ground cinnamon, and whole wheat flour.
2. Coat a griddle with cooking spray and preheat over medium heat. Drop a heaping tablespoon of batter onto the griddle, and heat for 4 minutes on one side.
3. Flip and heat for another 3 minutes on the other side. Respray griddle for each new set of pancakes.
4. Serve 5 pancakes topped with 2 tablespoons light maple syrup.
5. If you don't like the flavor of orange, you can substitute lemon or lime zest or eliminate the zest altogether; the pancakes are scrumptious either way.
6. If you don't serve all portions immediately, store in the refrigerator for up to 3 days or in the freezer in a tightly sealed plastic bag for up to a month.

Nutrition Facts

Per Serving: 209 calories, 11 g protein, 27 g carbohydrate, 7 g fat, 3 g saturated fat, 295 mg sodium, 126 mg cholesterol, 2 g fiber, 173 mg calcium

Breakfast

Chapter 7

Your Anti-Aging Recipes

Crunchy Banana Pop

Serves 2

Ingredients

½ cup unsweetened shredded wheat cereal
2 whole fresh bananas, peeled
2 kabob skewers or popsicle sticks (if desired)
½ cup low fat fruit flavored yogurt
2 tablespoons chopped peanuts (split)

Directions

1. Finely crush the cereal between two sheets of waxed paper.

2. Use two kabob skewers or popsicle sticks, and skewer two whole bananas through the end of the banana.

3. Spread half of the yogurt on each banana and roll in crushed cereal to coat, then roll each banana in half of the chopped peanuts.

4. Lay bananas on a cookie sheet or foil and freeze for at least two hours until firm.

Nutrition Facts

Per Serving: 301 calories, 10 g protein, 48 g carbohydrate, 11 g fat, 2 g saturated fat, 95 mg sodium, 2 mg cholesterol, 6 g fiber, 113 mg calcium

Breakfast

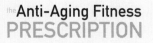

the **Anti-Aging Fitness**
PRESCRIPTION

Feta Broccoli Frittata

Serves 2

Ingredients

2 cups fresh or frozen broccoli florets
Olive oil flavored cooking spray
Two whole eggs (try eggs rich in omega 3 fats such as Eggland's Best)
Four egg whites or ½ cup egg substitute
½ teaspoon no-salt seasoning
½ teaspoon ground black pepper
2 ounces or ½ cup crumbled reduced fat feta cheese

Directions

1. Microwave broccoli florets for two minutes.

2. Coat a glass bowl with olive oil flavored cooking spray.

3. In a separate bowl, whisk together the eggs and egg whites with the no-salt seasoning and pepper.

4. Pour into prepared glass bowl, crumble feta cheese over the mixture and top with the broccoli.

5. Microwave for 90 seconds. Remove bowl, stir, and microwave for another 90 seconds.

Nutrition Facts

Per Serving: 199 calories, 22 g protein, 8 g carbohydrate, 9 g fat, 4 g saturated fat, 611 mg sodium, 221 mg cholesterol, 3 g fiber, 155 mg calcium

Breakfast

Chapter 7

Your Anti-Aging Recipes

Filo Ricotta Crisps

Serves 2

Ingredients

Cooking spray
1 teaspoon canola oil
⅛ cup chopped shallot (two small shallots)
One 15 ounce container low fat ricotta cheese
One ounce Roquefort or crumbled blue cheese
½ teaspoon no-salt seasoning
¼ teaspoon ground black pepper
Frozen filo dough (this recipe uses about ¼ of a one pound box)

Directions

1 Preheat oven to 450°F.

2 Coat a small saucepan with cooking spray and heat over medium heat with canola oil. Chop shallot and heat in saucepan until tender.

3 In a bowl, combine the ricotta cheese, crumbled Roquefort cheese, no-salt seasoning, ground black pepper, and cooked shallot.

4 Lay out two stacks of 4 pieces each of filo dough. Slice stacks lengthwise making 4 long strips, about 4 inches by 12 inches, then slice each long strip horizontally into 4 equal sections. Freeze remaining dough.

5 Spray a spoon with nonstick cooking spray to make it easier to drop the ricotta mixture. Spoon about 1 tablespoon ricotta mixture into one section of filo dough, fold up like you would fold a flag, and pinch edges to close.

6 Place onto a baking sheet coated with cooking spray. Bake for about 11 minutes or until golden brown. Store extra serving in refrigerator for up to 3 days; reheat (turn upside down to brown bottom side which will be soggy after storing) by baking at 200 degrees for 4 to 5 minutes.

Nutrition Facts

Per Serving: 342 calories, 29 g protein, 22 g carbohydrate, 18 g fat, 10 g saturated fat, 861 mg sodium, 81 mg cholesterol, 0 g fiber, 614 mg calcium

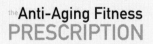

Festival of Fruit Salad

Serves 4

Ingredients

Two 11 ounce cans mandarin oranges packed in water or juice
¼ cup dried, sweetened cranberries
¼ cup walnuts, crushed
2 tablespoons shredded coconut

Directions

1 Combine all ingredients. Keep refrigerated.

Nutrition Facts

Per Serving: 139 calories, 3 g protein, 23 g carbohydrate, 5 g fat, 1 g saturated fat, 8 mg sodium, 0 mg cholesterol, 2 g fiber

Breakfast

107

Chapter 7

Your Anti-Aging Recipes

Tropical Cereal

Serves 1

Ingredients

1 cup low fat plain yogurt
¾ cup high fiber cereal, 100 calories worth such as Kashi Good Friends
   cereal
½ cup mandarin oranges packed in juice or water, drained
½ cup pineapple chunks packed in juice or water, drained
2 tablespoons slivered almonds

Directions

1 In a bowl, top yogurt with cereal, mandarin oranges, pineapple
chunks, and slivered almonds.

Nutrition Facts

*Per Serving: 412 calories, 18 g protein, 72 g carbohydrate, 9 g fat, 3 g
   saturated fat, 258 mg sodium, 15 mg cholesterol, 11 g fiber, 485 mg
   calcium*

Breakfast

Very Berry Smoothie

Serves 1

Ingredients

1 cup fresh or frozen, unsweetened berries such as raspberries, black-
berries or strawberries
1 cup plain low fat yogurt
4 ounces tofu, any style (look for calcium sulfate in the ingredients)
1 teaspoon granulated sugar
½ teaspoon pure vanilla extract or almond extract

Directions

1 Blend all ingredients with a blender or hand mixer. Add ice cubes
one at a time until you reach desired consistency.

Nutrition Facts

*Per Serving: 285 calories, 23 g protein, 28 g carbohydrate, 9 g fat, 3 g
saturated fat, 182 mg sodium, 15 mg cholesterol, 9 g fiber, 660 mg
calcium*

Breakfast

Chapter 7

**Your Anti-Aging
Recipes**

Lime Peanut Salad

Serves 2

Ingredients

6 scallions
1 ½ cups green cabbage, chopped
1 ½ cups red cabbage, chopped
1 cup shredded carrot
½ cup peanuts

For salad dressing:

¼ cup peanut butter
3 tablespoons white wine vinegar
1 tablespoon reduced sodium soy sauce
2 teaspoons brown sugar
1 clove garlic, minced
2 shakes of cayenne pepper

Directions

1 Chop scallions very thinly.

2 Toss scallions with green and red cabbage and shredded carrots.

3 Divide salad into two portions and top each salad with ¼ cup peanuts.

4 Whisk together salad dressing ingredients and dress each salad with half of the salad dressing. If you're saving half of salad to serve later, dress with peanuts and salad dressing immediately before serving.

Nutrition Facts

Per Serving: 489 calories, 17 g protein, 30 g carbohydrate, 37 g fat, 6 g saturated fat, 852 mg sodium, 0 mg cholesterol, 9 g fiber

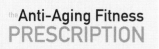

Pasta Primavera

Serves 2

Ingredients

¾ cup dry whole wheat pasta, any shape
Olive oil flavored cooking spray
1 tablespoon olive oil
½ cup chopped white or yellow onion
1½ cups broccoli florets, fresh or frozen (if frozen, cook in the
    microwave for 2 minutes)
1 cup sliced fresh or canned mushrooms, drained
1 cup spaghetti sauce
½ cup shredded mozzarella cheese

Directions

1. Heat one quart water to boiling, add pasta, and cook for 10 to 12 minutes.

2. Coat a large skillet with cooking spray, add 1 tablespoon olive oil, and sauté onion for 3 minutes.

3. Add broccoli florets and sliced mushrooms and heat for five minutes, stirring occasionally.

4. Add pasta to the skillet. Once pasta has heated through, remove pasta mixture from skillet and split into two servings.

5. Top each serving with ½ cup spaghetti sauce and sprinkle with ¼ cup shredded mozzarella cheese. Warm in the microwave for one minute to melt the cheese.

Nutrition Facts

Per Serving: 403 calories, 18 g protein, 56 g carbohydrate, 16 g fat, 6 g saturated fat, 724 mg sodium, 20 mg cholesterol, 6 g fiber, 283 mg calcium

Entrees —
Lunches or
Dinners

111

Chapter 7

**Your Anti-Aging
Recipes**

Caesar Shrimp Salad

Serves 2

Ingredients

4 tablespoons light Caesar dressing
1 tablespoon lemon juice
Ground black pepper
Cooking spray
6 ounces shrimp, tails removed and deveined
4 cups romaine lettuce, shredded
1 each yellow pepper and green pepper, thinly sliced
1 cup seasoned croutons
rice vinegar (if desired)

Directions

1 Whisk together 4 tablespoons light Caesar salad dressing, 1 table-spoon lemon juice, and a few shakes of black pepper.

2 Toss 12 large shrimp in dressing.

3 Coat a nonstick saucepan with cooking spray and sauté over medium heat for 3 minutes on each side or until shrimp turns pink. Set aside and let cool.

4 In a separate bowl, toss romaine lettuce, yellow pepper, and green pepper together, and top with shrimp. Add ½ cup seasoned croutons and sprinkle salad with a few shakes of rice vinegar if desired.

5 Divide into two portions and serve.

Nutrition Facts

Per Serving: 276 calories, 23 g protein, 24 g carbohydrate, 10 g fat, 2 g saturated fat, 580 mg sodium, 131 mg cholesterol, 6 g fiber

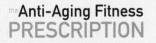

Chili

Serves 6

Ingredients

Olive oil flavored cooking spray
1 cup onion, chopped
1½ cups green pepper, chopped
One 16 ounce can red kidney beans
One 16 ounce can black beans
One 24 ounce can stewed tomatoes
¾ cup balsamic vinegar
1 tablespoon chili powder
1 teaspoon ground cumin powder
1 teaspoon onion powder
One 26 ounce jar spaghetti sauce
1 tablespoon minced garlic
1 pound cooked chicken breast meat, chopped into 1 inch cubes (or 1
    pound crumbled cooked ground turkey breast or ground chicken
    breast meat)

Directions

1 Coat a saucepan with cooking spray and heat over medium. Sauté
    onions and green pepper for 5 minutes, then turn down heat to low.

2 Rinse canned beans and stewed tomatoes in a colander to remove
    some of the sodium.

3 Add beans, tomatoes, and all remaining ingredients to saucepan and
    simmer for 20 minutes over low to medium heat.

4 Label and freeze in individual-sized portions for easy reheating.
    Defrost in refrigerator the night before serving.

Nutrition Facts

*Per Serving: 313 calories, 28 g protein, 44 g carbohydrate, 2 g fat, 0 g
    saturated fat, 500 mg sodium, 44 mg cholesterol, 12 g fiber*

Tasty Turkey Burgers

Serves 4

Ingredients

One pound ground turkey breast meat
¼ cup barbeque sauce
¾ cup water
⅓ cup seasoned breadcrumbs
2 teaspoons no-salt seasoning
¾ cup white onion, chopped
Cooking spray

Directions

1 Combine all ingredients in a medium-sized bowl.

2 Form into 4 patties.

3 Coat a saucepan with cooking spray. Cook over low to medium heat in a nonstick saucepan until cooked through.

Variation

Make meatballs using the same recipe. Fill a frying pan with about 1 inch water, form medium-size meatballs from the mixture, cover the pan (leave a little space for steam to escape) and "poach" the meatballs over medium heat until cooked through.

Nutrition Facts

Per Serving: 179 calories, 28 g protein, 13 g carbohydrate, 2 g fat, 1 g saturated fat, 446 mg sodium, 45 mg cholesterol, 1 g fiber

Fast Falafel

Serves 1

Ingredients

¼ cup falafel mix such as Manishevitz, Fantastic Foods, or Casbah
1 tablespoon canola oil
½ cup low fat plain yogurt
¼ cup cucumber, finely chopped
¼ cup fat free sour cream
1 tablespoon white onion, minced
1 teaspoon parsley, chopped
One 6 inch whole wheat pita bread
1 cup fresh baby spinach leaves
1 tomato, sliced

Directions

1. Prepare falafel mix according to package directions and pan fry in 1 tablespoon oil.

2. Make cucumber yogurt dressing by combining the next five in-gredients. The dressing is best made in advance and chilled in the refrigerator for at least one hour, but you can whip it up and serve immediately in a pinch.

3. Split open the pita bread and fill with cucumber yogurt dressing, spinach, tomato, and prepared falafel.

Nutrition Facts

Per Serving: 509 calories, 28 g protein, 72 g carbohydrate, 18 g fat, 2 g saturated fat, 1090 mg sodium, 13 mg cholesterol, 14 g fiber, 459 mg calcium

Spring Green Walnut Salad

Serves 2

Ingredients

4 cups mixed baby greens (spring mix, arugula, or baby spinach leaves)
1 cup mandarin oranges packed in juice, drained
4 tablespoons walnuts, chopped
4 tablespoons raspberry or balsamic vinaigrette salad dressing
1½ cups fresh raspberries

Directions

1 In a bowl, combine the first four ingredients and toss well.

2 Divide into two bowls, top each bowl with half of the raspberries, and serve.

Nutrition Facts

Per Serving: 234 calories, 7 g protein, 24 g carbohydrate, 14 g fat, 1 g saturated fat, 300 mg sodium, 0 mg cholesterol, 12 g fiber

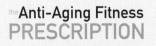

Pizza with Roasted Vegetables

Serves 4

Ingredients

Cooking spray
1 cup eggplant
1 red pepper
½ green pepper
¾ teaspoon no-salt seasoning
1½ tablespoons olive oil
1 large Neapolitan-style pizza crust
¼ cup sliced black olives, drained

Directions

1. Preheat the oven to 350° F. Coat a baking sheet with nonstick spray.

2. Thinly slice the eggplant and peppers.

3. Lay vegetables on the baking sheet and drizzle with olive oil, then sprinkle with no-salt seasoning. This will look like too many vegetables but after baking, they will shrink a bit.

4. Roast vegetables in the oven for 7 to 10 minutes and remove.

5. Turn up heat to 410° F. Top pizza crust with vegetables and sliced olives and bake for about 14 to 16 minutes, or until crust reaches desired crispness.

Nutrition Facts

Per Serving: 334 calories, 8 g protein, 55 g carbohydrate, 9 g fat, 1 g saturated fat, 121 mg sodium, 0 mg cholesterol, 4 g fiber

Chapter 7

**Your Anti-Aging
Recipes**

Chicken Curry

Serves 2

Ingredients

Cooking spray
½ cup yellow onion, chopped
½ teaspoon curry powder
1 cup fat free evaporated milk
2 tablespoons shredded coconut
4 tablespoons tomato paste
1 cup fresh or canned no salt added diced tomatoes, drained
8 ounces cubed raw chicken breast
3 cups fresh baby spinach leaves
½ teaspoon no-salt seasoning
1 cup cooked brown rice

Directions

1. Coat a skillet with cooking spray and heat over medium heat. Add chopped yellow onion and cook for about 7 to 9 minutes until soft.

2. Add curry powder and cook for one minute.

3. Stir in evaporated milk, shredded coconut, tomato paste, and diced tomato. Continue cooking and stir until mixture thickens, about 3 to 5 minutes.

4. Add cubed raw chicken breast, stirring occasionally and cook for another 5 minutes.

5. Add baby spinach leaves and no-salt seasoning, and cook for another 3 minutes, stirring occasionally.

6. Serve over rice.

Nutrition Facts

Per Serving: 434 calories, 35 g protein, 45 g carbohydrate, 5 g fat, 2 g saturated fat, 468 mg sodium, 66 mg cholesterol, 10 g fiber, 419 mg calcium

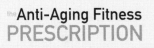
the **Anti-Aging Fitness**
PRESCRIPTION

Grapefruit Salad with Salmon

Serves 2

Ingredients

4 cups mixed baby greens
1 grapefruit, peeled and separated
1 small shallot, chopped
1 tablespoon canola oil
4 tablespoons balsamic vinaigrette dressing
3 ounces smoked salmon

Directions

1. Heat the canola oil in a saucepan, add the chopped shallot and sauté for 5 to 7 minutes.

2. In a separate bowl, combine all ingredients including shallot, and top with sliced lox and the dressing.

3. Divide into two bowls and serve.

Nutrition Facts

Per Serving: 204 calories, 10 g protein, 20 g carbohydrate, 11 g fat, 1 g aturated fat, 730 mg sodium, 10 mg cholesterol, 3 g fiber

Entrees —
Lunches or
Dinners

Chapter 7

**Your Anti-Aging
Recipes**

Turkey Empanadas with Low Sodium Salsa

Serves 2 (Makes 2 empanadas per serving)

Ingredients

2 tablespoons golden raisins
2 teaspoons cider vinegar
¼ cup white onion, chopped
1 clove garlic, minced
8 ounces raw ground turkey breast
¾ cup low sodium chicken broth
½ cup salsa for recipe plus ¾ cup salsa to top empanadas before serving
    (use Trader Joe's low sodium salsa or make your own with one 14½
    ounce can chopped no salt added tomatoes, ½ cup chopped cilantro,
    1 teaspoon olive oil, 2 tablespoons red wine vinegar, ¼ cup minced
    onion and 1 minced jalapeno pepper if desired)
1 tablespoon brown sugar
1 tablespoon slivered almonds
¼ teaspoon ground cinnamon
6 ounces raw whole grain bread dough (refrigerated or frozen, check
    the label for at least 2 grams of fiber per serving. In a pinch, you
    can use pizza dough)
1 egg
Cooking spray

Directions

1 Preheat the oven to 375° F.

2 Scoop golden raisins into a bowl, top with cider vinegar, and allow raisins to soak for 10 minutes.

3 Coat a skillet with cooking spray and heat over medium heat. Sauté ¼ cup chopped white onion with garlic for 2 minutes.

4 Turn down heat to low, add ground turkey breast, and cook for 4 minutes or until turkey is fully cooked.

5 Turn down heat to simmer, combine chicken broth with vinegar/raisin mixture, salsa, brown sugar, slivered almonds, and ground cinnamon.

6 Add chicken broth mixture to the pan, turn up heat, and bring to a boil for 2 minutes. Turn off heat.

7 Flour hands to handle bread dough, divide bread dough into four balls, roll out each ball to about 3 inches diameter.

8 Scoop one quarter of the mixture into each circle. Pinch up edges of dough to close and pierce dough 3 to 4 times with a fork, and place all six empanadas on a baking sheet coated with cooking spray.

9 Beat one egg, and brush the egg over the raw dough (you'll use about one half of the egg, discard remainder) and bake for 20 minutes.

10 Serve each empanada topped with 2 tablespoons salsa.

Nutrition Facts

Per Serving: 511 calories, 38 g protein, 70 g carbohydrate, 9 g fat, 1 g saturated fat, 599 mg sodium, 100 mg cholesterol, 3 g fiber

Entrees — Lunches or Dinners

Lemon Lime Salmon with Asparagus

Serves 2

Ingredients

Cooking spray
8 ounces raw salmon steak
1 fresh lemon
1 fresh lime
2 teaspoons olive oil
20 spears fresh or frozen asparagus

Directions

1. Preheat the oven to 350° F.

2. Coat a baking pan with cooking spray and place salmon steak on the pan.

3. Slice lemon and lime in half, squeeze juice from each over the salmon. Drizzle with the olive oil.

4. Bake for 22 to 25 minutes.

5. Add about ⅓ cup water to a frying pan, heat over medium until water begins to boil. Turn down heat to simmer, add asparagus, and cover, leaving top slightly open.

6. Simmer for 12 to 14 minutes, check water and add 2 tablespoons at a time as needed during cooking.

7. Drain water, divide and portion asparagus on plates, add half of salmon to asparagus.

8. Top each portion of asparagus with 2 tablespoons grated Parmesan cheese, and heat in the microwave for 45 seconds or until cheese begins to melt.

9. When reheating a leftover portion, sprinkle a little lime and lemon juice over asparagus and fish before heating to enhance flavor.

Nutrition Facts

Per Serving: 234 calories, 25 g protein, 9 g carbohydrate, 12 g fat, 2 g saturated fat, 51 mg sodium, 60 mg cholesterol, 3 g fiber

122

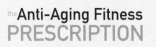

the**Anti-Aging Fitness**
PRESCRIPTION

Asian Mixed Green Salad

Serves 2

Ingredients

4 cups spring mixed greens or arugula
20 grape tomatoes, washed and halved
10 baby carrots, sliced
1 cup mandarin oranges (packed in juice), drained or 2 large ripe persimmons cut into quarters and spread apart
6 ounces roasted chicken cut into strips (to save time, use 6 ounces sliced deli chicken breast)
6 tablespoons raspberry vinaigrette salad dressing
1 cup sai fun or bean threads (dry cellophane noodles)

Directions

1 Divide greens, tomatoes, carrots, mandarin oranges, or persimmons between two bowls.

2 Top each serving with half of the chicken, dressing, and bean threads.

Nutrition Facts for Salad with Mandarin Oranges

Per Serving: 309 calories, 29 g protein, 37 g carbohydrate, 5 g fat, 1 g saturated fat, 758 mg sodium, 75 mg cholesterol, 4 g fiber

Nutrition Facts for Salad with Persimmons

Per Serving: 369 calories, 30 g protein, 54 g carbohydrate, 5 g fat, 1 g saturated fat, 754 mg sodium, 75 mg cholesterol, 5 g fiber

123

Chapter 7

Your Anti-Aging Recipes

Stoplight Pasta

Serves 2

Ingredients

¾ cup dry whole wheat pasta
1½ cups cut leaf frozen spinach
⅔ cup low fat ricotta cheese
1 clove garlic, minced
½ cup jarred roasted red peppers, chopped

Directions

1. Heat 1 quart water to boiling and add pasta, cook for 10 to 12 minutes.

2. Cook frozen spinach in the microwave, set aside.

3. In a bowl, combine low fat ricotta cheese, garlic, and roasted red peppers, and add to the pasta.

4. Fold in cooked spinach and combine with pasta mixture. Heat in microwave for 1 to 2 minutes to warm.

5. Divide into two portions and serve.

Nutrition Facts

Per Serving: 255 calories, 20 g protein, 39 g carbohydrate, 6 g fat, 3 g saturated fat, 770 mg sodium, 27 mg cholesterol, 7 g fiber, 358 mg calcium

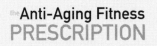

Glazed Pork and Apples

Serves 1

Ingredients

For the glaze:

3 tablespoons light pancake syrup
1 teaspoon Dijon mustard
1/8 teaspoon no-salt seasoning
1/8 teaspoon ground black pepper

For the main dish:

1 yellow apple, chopped
3 ounce pork loin cutlet or boneless pork chop
2 tablespoons plain bread crumbs
Cooking spray
1 teaspoon olive oil
3 tablespoons apple juice

Directions

1 In a bowl, combine light pancake syrup, Dijon mustard, no-salt seasoning, and pepper to make the glaze.

2 Chop yellow apple and set aside.

3 In a brown lunch bag add 2 tablespoons plain bread crumbs and the 3 ounce pork loin cutlet (or boneless pork chop), shake to coat.

4 Coat a skillet with cooking spray, add olive oil and heat over medium heat.

5 Cook pork for 2 minutes on each side. Add sliced apple and 3 tablespoons apple juice to the pan and bring to a boil.

6 Turn down the heat to low, pour the glaze mixture, cover, and simmer for another 4 minutes.

Nutrition Facts
Per Serving: 341 calories, 21 g protein, 51 g carbohydrate, 6 g fat, 2 g saturated fat, 390 mg sodium, 47 mg cholesterol, 4 g fiber

Entrees —
Lunches or
Dinners

125

Chapter 7

Your Anti-Aging Recipes

Broccoli, Beef and Tomatoes

Serves 2

Ingredients

3 cups fresh or frozen broccoli florets
8 ounces raw boneless lean sirloin steak, trimmed of excess fat
½ teaspoon no-salt seasoning
Ground black pepper
Cooking spray
3 scallions, thinly sliced
¼ teaspoon garlic powder
1 pint grape tomatoes
½ cup spaghetti sauce

Directions

1 Microwave broccoli until cooked, about 2 to 3 minutes.

2 Slice steak into ½ inch strips and season with no-salt seasoning and a few sprinkles of ground black pepper.

3 Coat a large skillet with cooking spray and preheat over medium. Add scallions and sauté for 4 minutes.

4 Add sirloin strips and cook for 4 to 5 minutes, stirring occasionally.

5 Add broccoli and sprinkle ¼ teaspoon garlic powder over the mixture. Turn down heat to low and cook for two minutes.

6 Add 1 pint grape tomatoes and cook for another two minutes.

7 Divide into two portions, top each portion with half of spaghetti sauce, and serve.

Nutrition Facts

Per Serving: 376 calories, 37 g protein, 25 g carbohydrate, 16 g fat, 6 g saturated fat, 343 mg sodium, 76 mg cholesterol, 7 g fiber

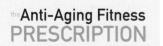

Chicken Mango Salad

Serves 2

Ingredients

Cooking spray
2 teaspoons olive oil
6 ounces raw chicken breast, sliced
15 ounce can no salt added diced tomatoes
1 tablespoon rice vinegar
2 tablespoons French salad dressing
4 cups spring greens or arugula
1 mango, peeled and sliced

Directions

1. Coat skillet with cooking spray and heat olive oil in a large skillet over medium heat.

2. Add sliced chicken breast and cook for 5 minutes, turning once.

3. Add the tomatoes (use liquid from the can) and bring to a boil, uncovered, for another 7 minutes.

4. Add rice vinegar and dressing to the skillet and mix thoroughly.

5. Serve the mixture over spring greens and slice the mango over the mixture, divide into two servings.

Nutrition Facts

Per Serving: 357 calories, 24 g protein, 51 g carbohydrate, 9 g fat, 1 g saturated fat, 288 mg sodium, 49 mg cholesterol, 8 g fiber

Chapter 7

Your Anti-Aging Recipes

Sweet and Sour Apricot Salsa Chicken

Serves 2

Ingredients

Cooking spray
Two 4 ounce chicken breasts
4 tablespoons all-purpose flour
Ground black pepper
2 tablespoons apricot jam
4 dried prunes, chopped
½ cup low sodium salsa (see recipe on page 120)
4 tablespoons white vinegar

Directions

1 Coat a skillet with cooking spray and heat over medium heat. Dredge the chicken breasts in the flour and lay in skillet. Sprinkle chicken with a few shakes of ground black pepper.

2 In a bowl, whisk together apricot jam, salsa, and white vinegar, and add the chopped prunes.

3 When chicken is cooked on one side, turn over and pour apricot salsa mixture over chicken, cover pan and turn down heat to low. Continue to simmer until chicken is cooked through.

Nutrition Facts

Per Serving: 301 calories, 29 g protein, 44 g carbohydrate, 2 g fat, 0 g saturated fat, 420 mg sodium, 66 mg cholesterol, 3 g fiber

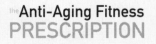

Scallops with Kumquat Chutney and Broccoli

Serves 2

Ingredients

For the chutney:

1 tablespoon canola oil
¼ cup red onion, finely chopped
⅛ teaspoon black or brown mustard seeds
⅛ teaspoon cumin
⅛ teaspoon tumeric
⅛ teaspoon ground cinnamon
14 fresh kumquats, peeled and sliced in half (remove any seeds) or ¾
    cup mandarin oranges packed in juice or water, drained
4 tablespoons brown sugar
1 tablespoon cooking sherry or cooking wine

For the main dish:

Cooking spray
1 broccoli florets, fresh or frozen
6 ounces scallops
1 cup cooked orzo
⅓ cup low sodium chicken broth

Chapter 7

**Your Anti-Aging
Recipes**

Directions

1. For the chutney, in a small saucepan, heat canola oil over medium heat. Add chopped onion, heat for 2 to 3 minutes.

2. Add the next four ingredients and heat for another 2 minutes.

3. Add kumquats or mandarin oranges and heat for 3 minutes.

4. Turn down the heat to simmer, add brown sugar and sherry and cover the pan, simmer for 6 minutes.

5. Uncover the pan and continue to simmer for 5 minutes to allow mixture to thicken.

6. Coat a skillet with cooking spray and heat over medium heat. Add broccoli and stir frequently for 2 to 3 minutes.

7. Add scallops and cook for 3 to 4 minutes, stirring frequently. Add orzo and chicken broth, heat, and stir mixture for another minute.

8. Divide into two portions and top each portion with one half of kumquat chutney.

Nutrition Facts

Per Serving: 461 calories, 22 g protein, 68 g carbohydrate, 12 g fat, 1 g saturated fat, 510 mg sodium, 27 mg cholesterol, 11 g fiber

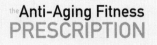
the Anti-Aging Fitness
PRESCRIPTION

Crab Cakes

Serves 2

Ingredients

2 slices whole wheat bread, crumbled into small pieces
2 eggs
1 tablespoon light mayonnaise
¼ cup yellow onion, chopped
½ teaspoon Old Bay seasoning
12 ounces fresh or canned lump crabmeat
Cooking spray
2 tablespoons canola oil

Directions

1 In a bowl combine the bread and eggs.

2 Add mayonnaise, yellow onion, and Old Bay seasoning. Finally, add lump crabmeat.

3 Form into nine 2 inch patties, and refrigerate for 30 minutes.

4 Coat a large skillet with cooking spray and heat over medium heat. Make the crab cakes in two batches, adding 1 tablespoon canola oil for each of two batches in the skillet.

5 Cook the crab cakes on each side for 2 to 3 minutes or until lightly browned.

Nutrition Facts

Per Serving: 418 calories, 317 g protein, 21 g carbohydrate, 21 g fat, 3 g saturated fat, 764 mg sodium, 241 mg cholesterol, 3 g fiber

Spreads

Serves about 4 (4 tablespoons per serving)

Ingredients

One 8 ounce container fat free sour cream
½ teaspoon vanilla extract or almond extract
½ teaspoon maple extract

Choose one to sweeten:

2 tablespoons jelly or jam or
1 tablespoon brown sugar or
1 tablespoon white sugar

Directions

1 Mix all ingredients together and store in the refrigerator.

Nutrition Facts with Jelly

Per Serving: 74 calories, 2 g protein, 6 g carbohydrate, 0 g fat, 0 g saturated fat, 93 mg sodium, 6 mg cholesterol, 0 g fiber, 81 mg calcium

Nutrition Facts with Brown or White Sugar

Per Serving: 57 calories, 2 g protein, 12 g carbohydrate, 0 g fat, 0 g saturated fat, 91 mg sodium, 6 mg cholesterol, 0 g fiber, 82 mg calcium

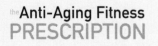

Peanutty Ricotta Spread

Makes about 6 servings (⅓ cup per serving)

Ingredients

One 15½ ounce container low fat ricotta cheese
3 tablespoons peanut butter
2 tablespoons honey (optional)

Directions

1 Mix all ingredients together and store in the refrigerator.

Nutrition Facts

*Per Serving: 142 calories, 11 g protein, 11 g carbohydrate, 8 g fat, 3 g
saturated fat, 223 mg sodium, 24 mg cholesterol, 0 g fiber, 187 mg
calcium*

Nutrition Facts without Honey

*Per Serving: 121 calories, 11 g protein, 5 g carbohydrate, 8 g fat, 3 g
saturated fat, 223 mg sodium, 24 mg cholesterol, 0 g fiber, 187 mg
calcium*

Spreads

Chapter 7

**Your Anti-Aging
Recipes**

Spreads

Spicy Pumpkin Dip

Serves 6 (about ½ cup per serving)

Ingredients

16 ounces canned pumpkin
⅓ cup brown sugar
2 teaspoons ground cinnamon
⅛ teaspoon ground cloves
¼ teaspoon ground nutmeg
½ teaspoon ground ginger
One 8 ounce container fat free sour cream

Directions

1 Combine all ingredients in a food processor and blend until smooth. Immediately refrigerate for up to 7 days, or freeze for up to 30 days.

2 Serve dip with graham crackers, toasted cinnamon or raisin bread, or mixed in a bowl with crunchy cereal.

Nutrition Facts

Per Serving: 90 calories, 2 g protein, 21 g carbohydrate, 0 g fat, 0 g saturated fat, 67 mg sodium, 0 mg cholesterol, 3 g fiber, 90 mg calcium

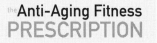

Creamy Tomato Soup

Serves 4

Ingredients

Two 10½ ounce cans low sodium tomato soup
16 ounces lowfat plain soymilk
1 teaspoon dried basil
4 tablespoons unsalted soy nuts

Directions

1. Mix first three ingredients in a large microwave-safe bowl.

2. Microwave for 3 to 4 minutes.

3. Divide into four soup bowls, and top each bowl with one tablespoon soy nuts.

Nutrition Facts

Per Serving: 188 calories, 7 g protein, 27 g carbohydrate, 5 g fat, 2 g saturated fat, 78 mg sodium, mg cholesterol, 3 g fiber

Baked Acorn Squash

Serves 2

Ingredients

1 acorn squash, halved
4 teaspoons brown sugar
1 teaspoon ground nutmeg
⅛ teaspoon ground cinnamon

Directions

1 Preheat the oven to 350° F.

2 Fill a small baking dish with ½ inch water. Scoop out any seeds and place acorn squash cut side down in the water and bake for 20 minutes.

3 In a small bowl, combine brown sugar, nutmeg and cinnamon.

4 Turn squash over and sprinkle half of the seasoning over each half and continue to bake, cut side up, for 20 minutes.

Nutrition Facts

Per Serving: 115 calories, 2 g protein, 21 g carbohydrate, 1 g fat, 0 g saturated fat, 9 mg sodium, 0 mg cholesterol, 4 g fiber

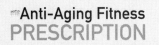

Tasty Greens

Serves 2

Ingredients

1 tablespoon olive oil
1 clove garlic, minced
2 cups collard, turnip, or mustard greens, fresh or frozen
1 teaspoon pepper
1 teaspoon no-salt seasoning
½ cup low sodium salsa (see recipe on page 120) (optional)

Directions

1. Heat oil in a skillet over medium heat until hot. Heat garlic until it begins to brown. Add greens and toss until thoroughly cooked. Then add pepper and no-salt seasoning and salsa, if desired. For a milder flavor, you can leave off the salsa.

Nutrition Facts

Per Serving: 95 calories, 2 g protein, 4 g carbohydrate, 7 g fat, 0 g saturated fat, 31 mg sodium, 0 mg cholesterol, 2 g fiber

Soups,
Sides and
Snacks

137

Chapter 7

**Your Anti-Aging
Recipes**

Layered Dip and Tortilla Chips

Serves 4

Ingredients

1 ripe avocado, mashed
1 cup fat free no salt added refried beans
1 cup low sodium salsa (see recipe on page 120)
1 cup fat free sour cream
4 ounces no salt added baked tortilla chips

Directions

1 Make a dip by layering the refried beans, salsa, and avocado.

2 Top with the sour cream.

3 Scoop the dip with the chips.

4 The avocado will turn brown overnight, so prepare right before eating.

Nutrition Facts

Per Serving: 267 calories, 8 g protein, 42 g carbohydrate, 8 g fat, 1 g saturated fat, 259 mg sodium, 6 mg cholesterol, 7 g fiber, 165 mg calcium

Black Bean Tomato Bruschetta

Serves 2 (1 baguette "boat" per serving)

Ingredients

One 17 inch whole wheat baguette
8 ounce can no salt added diced tomatoes, drained
8 ounce can black beans, rinsed and drained
Dried basil
3 tablespoons grated Parmesan cheese
Olive oil flavored cooking spray

Directions

1. Preheat the oven to 250° F.

2. Slice baguette in half lengthwise so you have two long baguette "boats."

3. Coat the bread with olive oil flavored cooking spray and toast on a cookie sheet in the oven for about 5 minutes.

4. Top each toasted bread section with half of the black beans and tomato and sprinkle half of the parmesan cheese and a shake of dried basil over each half.

Nutrition Facts

Per Serving: 388 calories, 20 g protein, 72 g carbohydrate, 4 g fat, 2 g saturated fat, 430 mg sodium, 7 mg cholesterol, 17 g fiber

Chapter 7

Your Anti-Aging Recipes

Roasted Chickpeas

Serves 2

Ingredients

19 ounce can chickpeas (also known as garbanzo beans)
Olive oil flavored cooking spray
¼ teaspoon dried oregano
⅛ teaspoon onion powder
⅛ teaspoon garlic powder
¼ teaspoon no-salt seasoning

Directions

1 Preheat the oven to 450° F.

2 Rinse the chickpeas for 2 to 3 minutes under cold water, drain and pat dry.

3 Coat a rimmed baking sheet with olive oil flavored cooking spray, and spread out chickpeas, spray with cooking spray and top with seasonings.

4 Bake for 30 minutes, stirring once halfway through baking.

Nutrition Facts

Per Serving: 288 calories, 12 g protein, 55 g carbohydrate, 3 g fat, 0 g saturated fat, 520 mg sodium, 0 mg cholesterol, 11 g fiber

Frozen Milk Pop

Serves 1

Ingredients

1 cup fat free milk
1 tablespoon chocolate syrup or 1 tablespoon powdered flavored drink
    mix

Directions

1 Mix milk with flavoring.

2 Pour into a paper cup with a popsicle stick (or use a coffee stirrer or
   drinking straw) and freeze for at least 2 hours.

Nutrition Facts

*Per Serving: 133 calories, 9 g protein, 25 g carbohydrate, 0 g fat, 0 g
    saturated fat, 120 mg sodium, 5 mg cholesterol, 0 g fiber, 223 mg
    calcium*

Desserts

Chapter 7

**Your Anti-Aging
Recipes**

Pudding Parfait

Serves 4

Ingredients

One 3.8 ounce package instant pudding, any flavor
2 cups fat free milk
12 tablespoons light dessert topping (such as Cool Whip Lite)
2 cups fresh berries, strawberries, raspberries, blackberries or blueberries

Directions

1 Make pudding according to package directions.

2 Separate into four portions and top each portion with ½ cup berries and 3 tablespoons light dessert topping. Use a clear parfait glass for a nice presentation.

Nutrition Facts

Per Serving: 184 calories, 5 g protein, 25 g carbohydrate, 2 g fat, 2 g saturated fat, 412 mg sodium, 2 mg cholesterol, 5 g fiber, 128 mg calcium

Creamy Chocolate Mousse

Serves 2

Ingredients

2 ounces sweetened, dark chocolate
1 cup light dessert topping (such as Cool Whip Lite)
1 cup low fat vanilla yogurt

Directions

1. Melt the chocolate in the microwave on half power for 1½ to 3 minutes.

2. Mix melted chocolate with the dessert topping and whip the mixture with a hand blender for 1 to 2 minutes.

3. Fold in the yogurt, blend, and pour into two dessert cups.

4. Refrigerate for one hour before serving.

Nutrition Facts

Per Serving: 338 calories, 8 g protein, 42 g carbohydrate, 15 g fat, 10 g saturated fat, 81 mg sodium, 10 mg cholesterol, 2 g fiber, 217 mg calcium

Desserts

Chapter 7

Your Anti-Aging Recipes

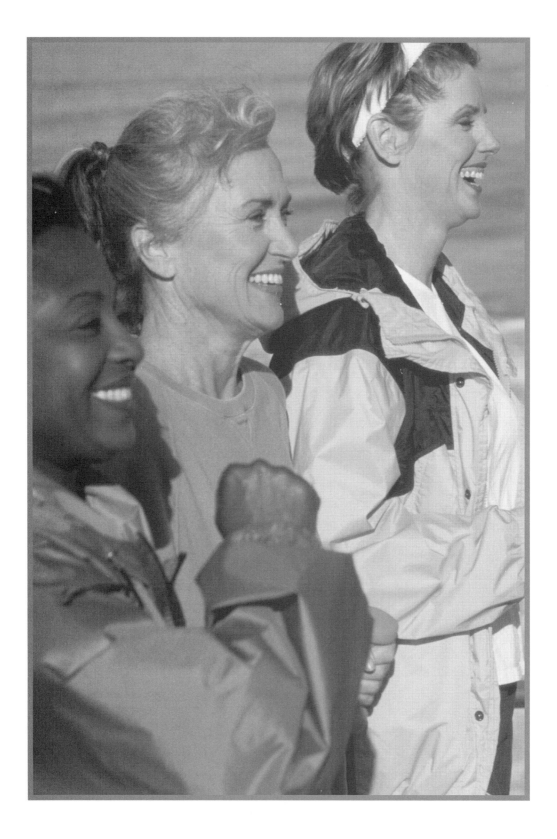

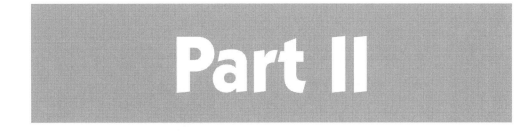

Your Eight-Week Anti-Aging Fitness Prescription

Your stepping stones to good health can be found right on these pages. Your measured plan begins with a little stretch, a short walk, and a serving of a vegetable every day. After the introduction, the pace picks up with the building phase, including more varied activity and one serving each of fruits, vegetables, and calcium-rich foods. At the end of the building phase you've worked up to a whole day's worth of balanced exercise and menu plans.

We know how tempting it is to jump ahead and incorporate all of these changes at once. But don't overdo it! New habits will stick around much longer if you approach them gradually. The new USDA food guide pyramid recommends small steps to achieve lifelong success with healthy eating and regular exercise.

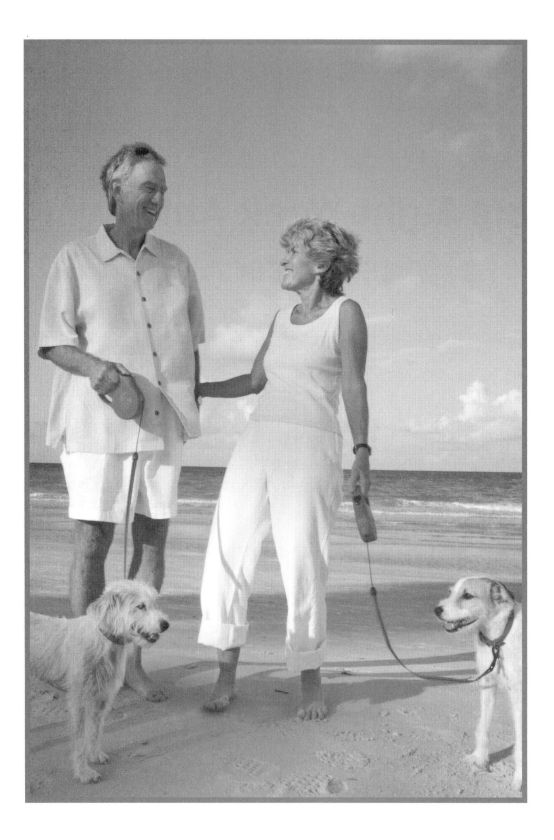

Before You Begin

How to Use the Activity Maps and Nutrition Diaries

Getting Started

FIRST STEP: GET A MEDICAL EVALUATION

Before you begin your Eight-Week Anti-Aging Fitness Prescription, you should get a thorough medical checkup with your physician. This way you get a baseline blood pressure, heart rate, and physical exam. Your doctor may also do a blood test to check such things like your cholesterol, blood sugar, and possibly a urinalysis and special tests such as a mammogram and bone density test based on your age, gender, and risk factors. If needed, your doctor can refer you to a medical specialist (such as another doctor, physical therapist, dietitian, occupational therapist) for specific medical concerns. You should also schedule routine visits with your dentist and dental hygienist and you should get periodic eye examinations. Seeing your doctor is the first step in improving and maintaining your health.

SECOND STEP: EVALUATE YOUR CURRENT CONDITION AND YOUR GOALS

Now that you are past the medical clearance and checkups, let's begin with your own home evaluation. Use the following guidelines in order to determine your ultimate success:

- Weigh yourself in the morning on a reliable bathroom scale (without clothes) before eating or drinking.
- Mark down your dress size (for women) or pant waist size (for men). Use a tape measure and measure the girth of your mid thigh. Now measure your mid upper arm. And measure your waist at the belly button.

- Mark down the areas(s) where you are experiencing pain (such as your left knee), if any. Then circle a number that describes your pain, with 10 being a trip to the emergency room, 5 being moderate pain, and 0 being no pain.
- Circle your typical energy level for daily activities, with number 10 being almost no energy to do anything, 5 as having moderate level of energy, and 1 as having excellent energy levels.
- Circle your typical daily stress levels, with 10 being uncontrolled severe stress, 5 as moderate stress that is annoying, and 1 being a very reasonable level of stress that you can control.
- Circle the number of hours you typically sleep at night.
- Record any other problem you would like to tackle during your Eight-Week Anti-Aging Fitness Prescription (such as smoking).

Now, record your goals for each of these measurements. You'll want to challenge yourself, but keep your goals realistic. You may be able to drop one dress size, for

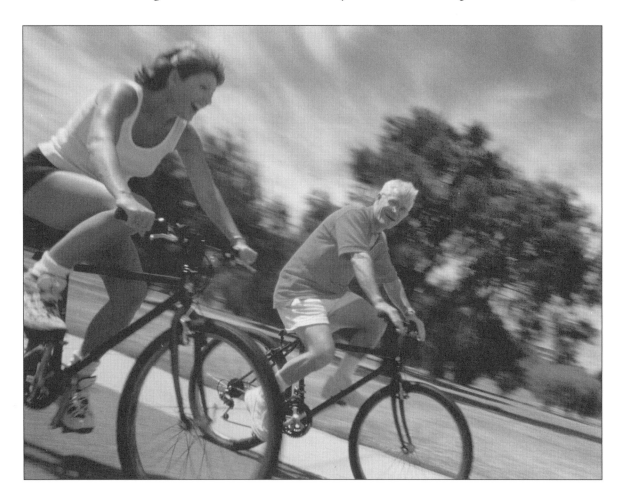

instance, but don't expect you'll be able to do more in just eight weeks. As a general rule of thumb, losing more than two pounds a week is considered unhealthy and is often unsustainable.

And, don't feel like you need to work on all of these measurements at once. If you're most concerned about your diet right now and your energy level is all right, then just focus on your diet. Again, the idea is to make gradual changes that you can stick with. After your eight weeks, you may find that your energy level has automatically improved with your diet changes. Or, you may want to go back to the beginning, this time focusing more upon your energy level.

YOUR CURRENT LEVEL	YOUR DESIRED GOALS	YOUR EIGHT-WEEK SUCCESS
1. Bodyweight (lbs): _____	1. Bodyweight (lbs): _____	1. Bodyweight (lbs): _____
2. Dress size: _____	2. Dress size: _____	2. Dress size: _____
3. Pants size: _____	3. Pants size: _____	3. Pants size: _____
4. Thigh girth (inches): _____	4. Thigh girth (inches): _____	4. Thigh girth (inches): _____
5. Arm girth (inches): _____	5. Arm girth (inches): _____	5. Arm girth (inches): _____
6. Waist girth (inches): _____	6. Waist girth (inches): _____	6. Waist girth (inches): _____
7. Pain level: 0 1 2 3 4 5 6 7 8 9 10 Pain Location: _____ Pain Location: _____	7. Pain level: 0 1 2 3 4 5 6 7 8 9 10 Pain Location: _____ Pain Location: _____	7. Pain level: 0 1 2 3 4 5 6 7 8 9 10 Pain Location: _____ Pain Location: _____
8. Energy level: 1 2 3 4 5 6 7 8 9 10	8. Energy level: 1 2 3 4 5 6 7 8 9 10	8. Energy level: 1 2 3 4 5 6 7 8 9 10
9. Stress level: 1 2 3 4 5 6 7 8 9 10	9. Stress level: 1 2 3 4 5 6 7 8 9 10	9. Stress level: 1 2 3 4 5 6 7 8 9 10
10. Sleep (hours): 4 5 6 7 8 9 10	10. Sleep (hours): 4 5 6 7 8 9 10	10. Sleep (hours): 4 5 6 7 8 9 10
11. Other: _____	11. Other: _____	11. Other: _____
12. Other: _____	12. Other: _____	12. Other: _____

THIRD STEP: SAY CHEESE

Go ahead and take a photo of yourself and place it in the appropriate box below. In 8 weeks you will take another photo of yourself and compare. If you follow the program you should be happy with your progress.

BEFORE   **Date:**_____

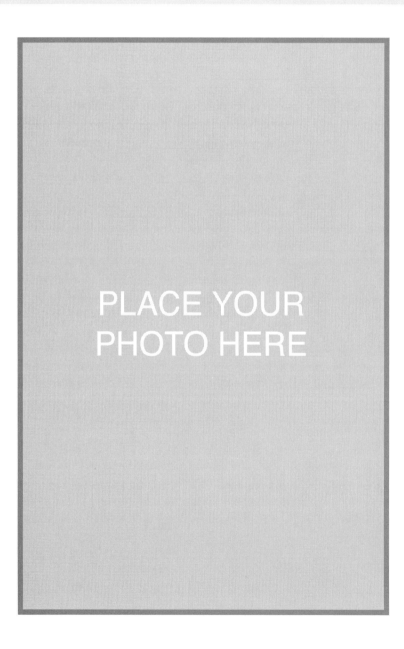

AFTER   **Date:**_____

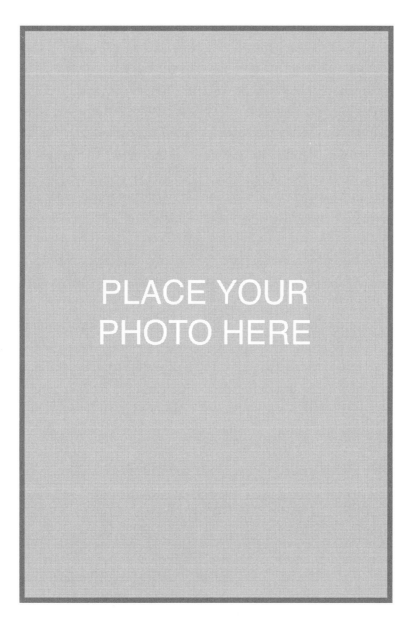

Your Activity Map

In the Eight-Week Anti-Aging Fitness Prescription that follows, you'll find an activity map for each day on which you can track your daily fitness pursuits on your handy activity map. Writing down your goals is a great way to get moving and stay moving. As we've learned, a combination of stretching along with aerobic and strength conditioning (including some balance exercises)—your Perfect Triangle Prescription—is optimal for anti-aging. As you can see from the at-a-glance program box that follows, the activity maps guide you day by day with a realistic plan to make these habits as routine as brushing your teeth—but not so routine as to become boring.

You start slow and easy with just 10 to 15 minutes of aerobic exercise 3 days a week and 1 set of simple strength-training exercises once a week during Phase 1. Then you gradually build through Phase 2 up to 5 days a week of more strenuous aerobic activity and 3 days a week of more advanced strength-training exercises. By Phase 3, you settle into a routine of 4 or 5 days of aerobics and 2 or 3 days of strength training that will keep you fit and feeling young for life!

Remember that this program is just a guide. If at any point you feel that you are not ready to progress to a new exercise or a new weight or duration as indicated, then don't. Conversely, if you ever feel that our recommendations are too easy, then pat yourself on the back and keep going just a little bit longer, or for a few more reps. Most importantly, listen to your body, watch your form to prevent injury, and don't overdo it. Refer back to the specific exercise chapters as often as you need to for guidelines on safe exercising proper form and read ahead for more details on how to keep your exercise at an intensity that is just right for you.

This is also your time to explore different activities and see what works for you and what doesn't. All of our daily workouts serve as a guide and not an absolute. So feel free to improvise a little here and there—incorporate plenty of variety to keep you from getting bored and to prevent injury and choose a program that naturally fits your personality, budget, and personal goals—but stick with the basic plan we outline for your weekly aerobic, strength, flexibility, and balance exercises.

Eight-Week Activity Map At a Glance

	DAY						
	1	Aerobic	Workouts:	Aerobic:	Strength:	Flexibility:	Balance:
	2	Warmup/Stretch	3 Aerobic	1) Time – 10 to 15 minutes	1) 1 set of 10 reps	1 set of 15	1 set of 15
Week 1	3	Aerobic	1 Strength	2) Intensity – OMNI RPE of 1 to 2	2) Intensity – OMNI RPE of 1 to 2	seconds	seconds
Phase 1	4	Strength	3 Warmup				
Introduction	5	Aerobic					
	6	Warmup/Stretch					
	7	Warmup/Stretch					
	8	Aerobic	Workouts:	Aerobic:	Strength:	Flexibility:	Balance:
	9	Strength	3 Aerobic	1) Time – 15 to 20 minutes	1) 1 set of 15 reps	1 set of 15	2 sets of 15
Week 2	10	Aerobic	2 Strength	2) Intensity – OMNI RPE of 2 to 3	2) Intensity – OMNI RPE of 2 to 3	seconds	seconds
Phase 2	11	Warmup/Stretch	2 Warmup				
Building	12	Strength					
	13	Aerobic					
	14	Warmup/Stretch					
	15	Aerobic	Workouts:	Aerobic:	Strength:	Flexibility:	Balance:
	16	Strength	4 Aerobic	1) Time – 20 to 25 minutes	1) 1 to 2 sets of 10 to 15 reps	1 set of 15 to	1 set of 30
Week 3	17	Aerobic	2 Strength	2) Intensity – OMNI RPE of 3 to 4	2) Intensity – OMNI RPE of 3 to 4	30 seconds	seconds
Phase 2	18	Aerobic	1 Warmup				
Building	19	Strength					
	20	Aerobic					
	21	Warmup/Stretch					
	22	Aerobic	Workouts:	Aerobic:	Strength:	Flexibility:	Balance:
	23	Strength	4 Aerobic	1) Time – 25 to 30 minutes	1) 1 to 2 sets of 8 to 12 reps	2 sets of 15 to	1 to 2 sets of
Week 4	24	Aerobic	2 Strength	2) Intensity – OMNI RPE of 4 to 5	2) Intensity – OMNI RPE of 4 to 5	30 seconds	30 seconds
Phase 2	25	Aerobic	1 Warmup				
Building	26	Strength					
	27	Aerobic					
	28	Warmup/Stretch					
	29	Aerobic	Workouts:	Aerobic:	Strength:	Flexibility:	Balance:
	30	Strength	5 Aerobic	1) Time – 30 to 40 minutes	1) 2 sets of 8 to 12 reps	2 sets of 15 to	1 to 2 sets of
Week 5	31	Aerobic	2 Strength	2) Intensity – OMNI RPE of 5 to 6	2) Intensity – OMNI RRPE of 5 to 6	30 seconds	30 to 60
Phase 2	32	Aerobic					seconds
Building	33	Strength					
	34	Aerobic					
	35	Aerobic					
	36	Aerobic	Workouts:	Aerobic:	Strength:	Flexibility:	Balance:
	37	Strength	4 Aerobic	1) Time – 30 to 45 minutes	1) 1 to 3 sets of 8 to 12 reps	2 to 3 sets of	2 to 3 sets of
Week 6	38	Aerobic	3 Strength	2) Intensity – OMNI RPE of 6 to 7	2) Intensity – OMNI RPE of 6 to 7	15 to 30	30 to 60
Phase 2	39	Aerobic				seconds	seconds
Building	40	Strength					
	41	Aerobic					
	42	Strength					

Eight–Week Activity Map At a Glance, cont.

	DAY		Workouts:	Aerobic:	Strength:	Flexibility:	Balance:
	43	Aerobic	5 Aerobic	1) Time – 30 to 45 minutes	1) 1 to 3 sets of 8 to 15 reps	1 to 3 sets of	1 to 3 sets of
	44	Strength	2 Strength	2) Intensity – OMNI RPE of 5 to 7	2) Intensity – OMNI RPE of 5 to 7	15 to 30	30 to 60
Week 7	45	Aerobic				seconds	seconds
Phase 3	46	Aerobic					
Maintenance	47	Strength					
	48	Aerobic					
	49	Aerobic					
	50	Aerobic	Workouts:	Aerobic:	Strength:	Flexibility:	Balance:
	51	Strength	4 Aerobic	1) Time – 30 to 45 minutes	1) 1 to 3 sets of 8 to 15 reps	1 to 3 sets of	1 to 3 sets of
Week 8	52	Aerobic	3 Strength	2) Intensity – OMNI RPE of 5 to 7	2) Intensity – OMNI RPE of 5 to 7	15 to 30	30 to 60
Phase 3	53	Aerobic				seconds	seconds
Maintenance	54	Strength					
	55	Aerobic					
	56	Strength					

CHOOSING YOUR EXERCISE INTENSITY

For the purposes of this book we want to keep your exercise program simple and safe, so we want you to focus on how you feel during all of your activity and exercise sessions. We understand that in the past you may have used other methods, such as target heart rate charts or graphs, a heart rate monitor, or manually checking your pulse, walking for a predetermined number of steps using a pedometer, or walking at a certain pace for a predetermined distance or time. All of these methods have their place and can be used in a variety of situations but in this program we want you to focus on how you feel during all of your activities and exercise sessions. As we noted earlier, it can be easy to overtrain simply because you're focused so much upon these goals rather than upon how you feel.

In order to help monitor your intensity (how hard you are working) during the pro-gram we want you to focus on using our 8-point Self-Monitoring Scale. Typically, the more experience the person has with activity, exercise, or sport, the more likely they have a good understanding how hard they can push themselves without injury. The Self-Monitoring Scale will assist both the novice and experienced reader in determining safe limits for exercise and activity sessions.

1. Train using your inner intensity gauge.

- **Aerobic** — select an intensity (how fast and how hard) during your aerobic exercises (such as walking, bicycling, dancing, playing tennis) that allows you to exercise hard enough while meeting all of the following key points: 1) use the talk test to gauge your aerobic exercises such as walking, biking, dancing, hiking. The talk test involves being able to carry on a conversation with a person next to you without gasping for air. Another technique is that you can sing a song if you wanted to (but you won't sing of course), 2) you use proper form and posture during the entire exercise, 3) you have no symptoms or pain.

- **Strength** — select an intensity (how much weight, difficulty of elastic resistance) during your strength exercises (such as dumbbell chest press, elastic pull to chest, sit to stand) that allows you to exercise hard enough while meeting all of the following key points: 1) you're able to perform in the range of 1 to 3 sets of 8 to 15 reps, 2) you use proper form and posture during the entire exercise, 3) you have no symptoms or pain, 4) you don't hold your breath during the exercises.
- **Stretching** — stretch to a point where you feel no pain at end range or limit of the stretching exercise. The stretches should feel as hard as when you yawn.
- **Balance** — select an intensity that allows you to able to keep your balance and stability in a safe manner without putting you at a risk for falling.

2. Train without pain.

Of course, you are going to experience a little discomfort and fatigue in your muscles during your aerobic and strength training exercises, but don't exercise to the point

where you feel severe fatigue, dizziness, loss of balance, nausea, headache, migraines, blurry vision, chest pain, difficulty breathing, upset stomach, numbness or tingling in your legs and arms, joint pain, or injury to your muscles and joints. If you experience these or any other unusual symptoms, see your physician.

3. Train without strain.

Don't hold your breath during exercise. As you recall, this places unnecessary pressure on your blood vessels.

4. Train according to your goals.

When you perform a task with a goal or purpose in mind then you usually get more out of it. So your goal for a particular workout might be to have some fun (play tennis), reduce your stress (blow off some steam after work), lose some weight, improve your performance for a sport (play better golf), get limber and flexible after sitting at work all day, or meet new people doing something active.

5. Train according to your medical needs.

You may have to modify certain aspects of your workout if you have arthritis, asthma, diabetes, osteoporosis, high blood pressure, heart disease, or other chronic conditions. We've included a Very Low Intensity Program for those of you who fit into this category, but be sure to consult your physician first.

6. Train with good form and technique.

By doing each exercise properly with controlled movements and good posture, you improve the effectiveness of the exercise and minimize injury.

7. Train with safety in mind.

Use proper sports equipment (such as a bicycle helmet) to prevent injury. Avoid exercises or sports that are beyond your current ability. Read and learn proper safety techniques for each exercise and activity you engage in.

8. Train for good health and fun.

Try to keep your fitness programs fun and enjoyable. Many of us have too much stress in our lives. We feel that activity, fitness, sports, and exercise should be a pursuit that enriches your life rather than being another dreaded workout you have to force your body through. This is why we recommend a variety of activities. If you are not experienced in a variety of activities then we recommend you take classes and challenge yourself.

Aerobic Training Intensity Scale

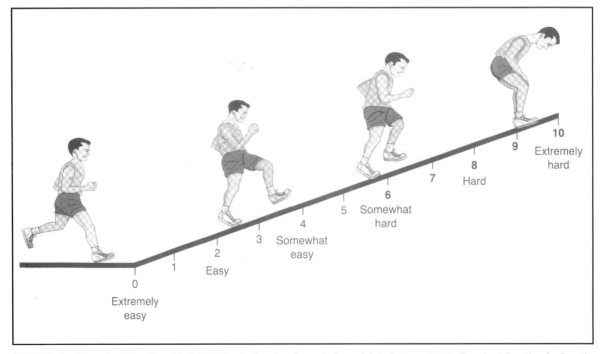

OMNI Scale of Perceived Exertion: Adult, Walking to Running Format . From R.J. Robertson, 2004, *Perceived Exertion for Practitioners: Rating Effort With the OMNI Picture System*, page 142. © 2004 by Robert J. Robertson. Reprinted with permission from Human Kinetics (Champaign, IL).

OMNI Ratings of Perceived Exertion (RPE) Scale

In addition to this Self-Monitoring Scale, a Ratings of Perceived Exertion (RPE) scale can be used to help you gauge how hard you should be working during your activity and exercise program. We have included a new RPE scale called the OMNI Perceived Exertion Scale using a picture system. The original RPE scale was developed by Gunnar Borg, PhD, currently professor emeritus of perception and psychophysics in Stockholm University. His system uses a number and word description for gauging exercise intensity. The new OMNI RPE scale was developed by Robert J. Robertson, PhD, a researcher at the University of Pittsburgh. The term OMNI is derived from the word omnibus, which means serving several purposes at once. This means the scale uses three ways (words, numbers, and pictures) to describe how hard a person is exerting themselves in terms of effort, strain, discomfort, and fatigue in a variety of activities such as walking and weight training.

There are two OMNI RPE scales used in this book — one for aerobic exercises, and one for strength exercises. Look at the person at the bottom of the scale. If you feel like this person when you are doing aerobic activity or strength training exercises, then your exertion will be extremely easy and

Strength Training Intensity Scale

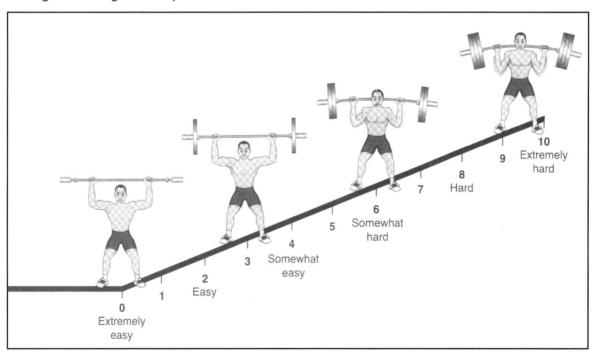

OMNI Resistance Exercise Scale: Adult. From R.J. Robertson, 2004, *Perceived Exertion for Practitioners: Rating Effort With the OMNI Picture System*, page 144. © 2004 by Robert J. Robertson. Reprinted with permission from Human Kinetics (Champaign, IL).

the number you select would be 0. Now look at the person at the top of each scale and if you feel like this person, then your exertion will be extremely hard and the number you select would be 10. If your exertion is somewhere in between these two ranges, then you would select a number between 0 and 10. For the purposes of this eight-week program, you will be working at an OMNI RPE of 1 to 2 for Phase 1, OMNI RPE ranging from 2 to 3 and up to 6 to 7 for Phase 2 and finally, tapering off at OMNI RPE of 5 to 7 for Phase 3.

Very Low Intensity Program

If you suffer from a chronic condition that makes most exercising difficult, are recovering from an illness, have marked pain in your joints, or are severely overweight, try this program instead of or before you start the Eight-Week Anti-Aging Fitness Prescription.

Warm up: Spend 1 to 3 minutes loosening up before exercise or activity.

- March in place (seated or standing)

- Shake, rattle and roll (seated or standing)

Aerobic: Start at 5 to 10 minutes and progress 2 minutes per week up to 15 to 30 minutes per session. Aim for 2 to 3 times per week. At this intensity, you shouldn't feel any pain and you should be able to sing a song. You don't have to sing, of course, but you should be able to. Please select one of the following activities for your aerobic activity session:

1. Outdoor walk

2. Indoor walk (such as a mall)

3. Stationary bike

4. Pool walking or exercises

Strength: Start at 1 set of 10 reps and progress to 1 to 2 sets of 10 reps per session. Start with 1 to 2 lbs weights or yellow or red exercise elastic. Aim for 1 to 2 times per week. Use an intensity that allows you to train with good form, no pain and breathe naturally. Try all of the following strength training exercises if your are able to perform them:

- Sit to stand squats

- Elastic pull to chest

- Dumbbell biceps curl

- Supine bridging

- Abdominal bracing

- Pelvic floor

Flexibility: Aim for 1 set of 10 to 15 seconds. Aim for 2 to 3 times per week. Stretch as hard as when you yawn. In other words, it's an easy stretch. Try all of the following flexibility exercises if you are able to perform them:

- Wrist stretches
- Neck stretches
- Hands behind back stretch
- Yawn stretch
- Calf stretch
- Hamstring stretch
- Inner hip stretch
- Outer hip stretch

Balance: Start at 1 to 2 seconds and progress as able to 10 seconds for 2 to 3 sets. Aim for 2 to 3 times per week. Perform the following balance exercise:

- Dancer's balance (modified)

Cool down: Spend 1 to 3 minutes gradually slowing down after exercise or activity with easy movements and gentle breathing techniques. Perform the following relaxation exercise:

- Diaphragmatic breathing

Sample activities: Very light chair and mat exercises, walking slowly at your natural speed, easy bicycling, gentle calisthenics, very light resistance training (weights or elastic), easy gardening, easy housework such as dusting.

Your Nutrition Diary

In the Eight-Week Anti-Aging Fitness Prescription that follows, you'll find a nutrition diary for each day on which you can record your food and drink intake. The nutrition diary is an important tool you can use to keep track of your eating habits and patterns, hunger level, and fruit and vegetable intake.

After the first three weeks, each day includes at least 3 servings of fruits and vegetables from different color groups. The Color Your World chart on page 162 will give you a guideline to different-colored fruits and vegetables. You may substitute fruits or vegetables within the color groups. If you don't like blueberries, you can have strawberries or any fruit from the red/purple group and if you wouldn't touch green peas, substitute a favored yellow/green group vegetable such as green beans. You may notice that some color groups have only fruits or only vegetables. This chart represents the well-researched phytochemicals and the food sources, and as research continues, it will expand to include more types of fruits and vegetables.

Drinks aren't always included in your meal plan but non-caloric drinks or very low-calorie drinks, including water, coffee, tea and flavored seltzer water are allowed. If you have coffee every morning, account for your add-ons (one teaspoon of sugar is 15 calories; one tablespoon of half-and-half is 20 calories and 1 gram of saturated fat). The calories can climb with each cup of coffee you prepare.

Each menu has about 1600 calories per day, 1200 mg calcium from calcium-rich foods and 3 different colored fruits and 3 different colored vegetables. We've reused ingredients as much as possible to overlap days and make shopping a snap. You can follow these anti-aging menus in the nutrition diaries, or you can plan your own well-rounded meals that begin with our anti-aging basics (see Mix 'n Match Anti-Aging Meal Plan below). If you're watching your calories, an estimate for calories is listed with each food group.

You may notice on the menus, beginning with day 22, that the percentage of calories from carbohydrate, fat and protein don't add up to 100%. There's a very good reason for this. For the purposes of this eating plan, we've used the standard estimate of 4 calories per gram of carbohydrate and protein and 9 calories per gram of fat. There are small variations to this calorie per gram estimate; sometimes the actual calories vary, such as 9.28 calories per gram of olive oil or 9.37 calories per gram of animal fat. The actual percentages are skewed by these small differences in the calorie counts. Rest assured that you are getting a very well balanced, nutritious plan regardless of this small variation in the percentages each day.

MIX 'N MATCH ANTI-AGING MEAL PLAN

You'll see that in the first few weeks of the program, we will not be asking you to change your whole diet, but simply to add a serving of vegetable (in Week 1), a serving of fruit (in Week 2), and a calcium-rich food (in Week 3) per day. By Week 4, though, when you are used to eating more of these key foods, we'll start giving you menu plans for the whole day. Each menu plan was put together following a simple mix 'n match plan. If you don't like any of the menu plans or want to try some new dishes, you can use these principles to stay on a healthy diet that gives you all the anti-aging nutrition you'll need for life! Choose your basic necessities (vegetables, fruits, and calcium-rich foods) first, then add choices from Wholesome Grains, the Finest Fats, and Lean, Mean Proteins.

THE BASIC NECESSITIES: VEGETABLES, FRUITS, AND CALCIUM-RICH FOODS

First, choose 3 different colored vegetables. Choose at least one serving of vegetables (½ cup cooked or 1 cup raw) from three different color groups, such as red, orange, and green (see the Color Your World chart on page 162). Vegetables provide about 25 calories per serving. The exceptions are starchy vegetables such as corn, lima beans, peas, and winter squash (acorn, butternut), which have 80 calories per half cup serving.

Second, choose 3 different colored fruits. Choose at least one serving of fruit (1 medium whole fruit, 1 cup berries or cut fruit, ¼ cup dried fruit, or ½ cup canned fruit) from three different color groups, such as red, yellow/green and orange (see Color Your World chart on page 162). Fruits provide about 60 calories per serving.

Third, choose 3 calcium-rich foods. Choose calcium-rich foods totaling at least 1,200 mg of calcium every day (see the Cool Calcium Choices chart on page 163). The recipes will fulfill some servings of carbohydrates, proteins and fats, so look for the nutrition facts for the recipe in Anti-Aging Recipes if you're keeping your calories in check.

You'll find produce in our menu plans that aren't listed in the Color Your World list. That doesn't mean you shouldn't eat them! The list includes fruits and vegetables containing phytochemicals that have been extensively studied by various researchers and whose specific health benefits we can prove. There are many phytochemicals in our diet that have not yet been thoroughly researched but have the potential to improve general health and prevent some chronic diseases. For example, the newly discovered phytochemcial N–coumaroyltyramine is found in bananas, which are conspicuously missing from this list. We don't know exactly what N–coumaroyltyramine does yet—it has been speculated to act as an anti-proliferation agent and as a neurotransmitter—but we know that bananas are good for you. While it's tempting to champion the well-researched fruits or vegetables over the others, every single fruit and vegetable offers you some health benefit.

Color Your World

Color Group	Provides	Benefits	Sources
Red	Lycopene	May reduce risk of prostate cancer and heart disease and can protect the cells in the body from oxidative damage.	Tomato sauce, tomato puree, tomato soup, tomato juice, tomatoes cooked and raw, pink grapefruit, pink grapefruit juice, and watermelon. (Processing enhances the bioavailability of lycopene, so choose no-salt canned versions.)
Red/Purple	Anthocyanins	May have a beneficial effect on heart disease by inhibiting blood clot formation and may help with age-related declines in mental function.	Red grapes, grape juice, prunes, plums, cranberries, red apples, blueberries, blackberries, strawberries, raspberries, cherries, purple cabbage, figs, purple passion fruit, pomegranate, cooked beets, cranberry juice, and cranberry sauce.
Orange	Alpha- and Beta-carotene	Protect against cancer by preventing oxidative damage and promote healthy vision.	Carrots, mangos, apricots, cantaloupes, pumpkin, acorn squash, winter squash, sweet potatoes, persimmons, butternut squash, yellow squash, orange pepper.
Orange/Yellow	Beta-cryptothanxin	Helps fight heart disease, decreases the risk for some cancers	Oranges, tangerines, tangelos, peaches, papayas, nectarines, pineapples, guava, kumquats, starfruit.
Yellow/Green	Lutein and zeaxanthin	May help reduce the risk of cataracts and age-related macular degeneration.	Arugula, spinach, collard greens, mustard greens, turnip greens, yellow corn, green peas, avocados, honeydew melon, kiwifruit, zucchini, romaine lettuce, green beans, green and yellow peppers.
Green	Sulforaphane, isothiocyanate, indoles	Broccoli may play an important role in decreasing the risk of premenopausal breast cancer. The green group is rich in vitamin K which is linked to improved bone health.	Broccoli, Brussels sprouts, cabbage, Chinese cabbage, bok choi, kale, watercress.
White/Green	Allyl sulfides, flavonoids (quercetin and kaempferol)	Protects against bacterial, viral, and fungal infections, lowers total blood cholesterol and LDL cholesterol, protects against some cancers.	Garlic, leeks, onions, shallots, celery, pears, endive, chives, asparagus, mushrooms

Food	Milligrams Calcium	Calories
Very Berry Smoothie Recipe	660 mg calcium	285 calories
Filo Ricotta Crisps Recipe	614 mg calcium	342 calories
Fast Falafel Recipe	459 mg calcium	509 calories
Tropical Cereal Recipe	485 mg calcium	412 calories
Yogurt Bowl Recipe	466 mg calcium	413 calories
1 cup plain nonfat yogurt	452 mg calcium	137 calories
1 cup plain lowfat yogurt	415 mg calcium	110 calories
1 cup fruit-flavored lowfat yogurt	372 mg calcium	250 calories
Stoplight Pasta Recipe	358 mg calcium	255 calories
2 ounces American cheese (processed)*	344 mg calcium	213 calories
Sweet Cottage Cheese Bowl Recipe	334 mg calcium	377 calories
1½ ounces Swiss cheese*	332 mg calcium	160 calories
1½ ounces mozzarella cheese*, part skim	328 mg calcium	107 calories
3 ounces sardines canned in oil	325 mg calcium	177 calories
1 cup 2% chocolate milk	285 mg calcium	180 calories
1 cup 1% buttermilk	284 mg calcium	98 calories
Pasta Primavera Recipe	283 mg calcium	403 calories
1 cup 2% milk	270 mg calcium	122 calories
1 cup 1% milk	264 mg calcium	102 calories
6 ounces Tropicana calcium-fortified orange juice (limit to 6 ounces per day, not for diabetics please)	263 mg calcium	83 calories
Fruit and Cheese Foldover Recipe	246 mg calcium	271 calories
1 cup fat-free milk	223 mg calcium	83 calories
Frozen Milk Pop Recipe	223 mg calcium	123 calories
Creamy Chocolate Mousse	217 mg calcium	338 calories
1 cup boiled soybeans	175 mg calcium	298 calories
Fluffy Orange Pancakes Recipe	173 mg calcium	209 calories
4 ounces firm tofu**	198 mg calcium	69 calories
1 cup cooked turnip greens	197 mg calcium	29 calories
Peanutty Ricotta Spread Recipe	187 mg calcium	121 calories
1 cup cooked Collard Greens	160 mg calcium	60 calories
Feta Broccoli Frittata Recipe	155 mg calcium	199 calories
½ cup nonfat frozen yogurt	138 mg calcium	80 calories
Pudding Parfait Recipe	128 mg calcium	184 calories
1 cup baked beans	127 mg calcium	236 calories
1 cup cooked kale	98 mg calcium	36 calories
1 cup cooked broccoli	62 mg calcium	55 calories
1 cup vegetarian refried beans	68 mg calcium	188 calories

*Choose once per day to control your intake of saturated fat, cholesterol and sodium.

**Calcium values are only for tofu processed with a calcium salt or calcium sulfate. Tofu processed with a non-calcium salt will not contain much calcium.

WHOLESOME CARBS

Choose 4 or more wholesome carbs. These carbohydrate choices provide 70 to 120 calories per serving. For breads, crackers and cereals, look for the words "whole grain" on the ingredients list and "trans-free" on the nutrition facts label. Look for at least 2 grams of fiber in one serving of bread, rice, pasta or crackers and for cereal, look for at least 3 grams of fiber and less than 5 grams of sugar in one serving.

Here's how to measure servings of carbs. One serving equals:
- ½ cup breakfast cereal
- 1 slice bread
- ½ whole grain bagel, 230 calories or less per bagel
- One 8" whole wheat soft tortilla
- One 6" whole wheat pita
- One whole grain English muffin
- One whole grain frozen waffle
- 3 ounces of potato with skin, any type
- ⅓ cup rice, cooked amount (use less of seasoning packet to reduce sodium)
- ½ cup whole wheat pasta, cooked amount

THE FINEST FATS

Choose 4 or more good (unsaturated) fats. These fats provide about 45 calories per serving:
- One tablespoon nuts, any type
- One tablespoon seeds, any type
- 5 olives, black or green (high sodium, limit to one serving per day)
- 1 tablespoon light, trans-free margarine spread
- ⅛ avocado
- 1 tablespoon salad dressing
- 1 tablespoon canola oil light mayonnaise
- 2 tablespoons light salad dressing
- 2 tablespoons hummus
- 1 teaspoon oil (choose from safflower, sunflower, olive)

LEAN, MEAN PROTEINS

Choose 6 or more servings. Each serving provides 40 to 60 calories. When choosing meats, look for 3 grams of fat per ounce or less. Whole eggs with omega-3 fats are widely available, these are eggs in the shell in a regular egg carton, and the carton label will have the words "omega-3." These eggs typically have a little less saturated fat (you save about 0.3 grams) than a standard egg and they provide 0.4 grams or more of omega-3 fatty acids. Whole eggs provide 75 calories per serving.

Here's how to measure servings of proteins. One serving equals:
- ¼ cup canned beans (high sodium, limit to 3 servings per day, always rinse and drain to remove some sodium)
- ¼ cup fat-free or 1% cottage cheese (choose lower sodium when possible)
- 1 ounce sliced turkey breast, lean roast beef, lean ham, chicken breast (choose lower sodium when possible)

- 1 ounce 90% lean ground beef, ground pork or ground turkey
- 1 ounce skinless chicken and turkey, both white and dark meat
- 1 ounce beef select or choice grades trimmed of fat, filet mignon, round, sirloin, flank steak, or tenderloin, T-bone or porterhouse steak; or rib, chuck, or rump roast.
- 1 ounce pork tenderloin, Canadian bacon or ham (high sodium, choose no more than one ounce per day), or pork center loin chop
- 1 ounce game: Duck or pheasant (no skin), venison, buffalo, or ostrich
- 1 egg (limit 5 whole eggs per week) or ¼ cup egg substitute or 2 egg whites

the Anti-Aging Fitness
PRESCRIPTION

Activity Map

Why Exercise?

- Sleep better.
- Reduce stress.
- Increase energy.
- Enhance mood.
- Improve posture.
- Boost immune system.
- Fight anxiety and depression.
- Reduce risk of certain types of cancer.
- Reduce risk of stroke, heart disease, diabetes, osteoporosis.
- Reduce memory decline.
- Help prevent injuries.
- Keep you independent during your lifetime.
- Control weight.
- Improve self-esteem.

From Z and Tracy: Welcome to your anti-aging lifestyle program. Of course you can start this program on any day but we would prefer if you read the book for a few days and wait until the first Monday to start. So ideally Day 1 should be a Monday. We look forward to working with you and guiding you through this fun and simple program. We'll be with you every step of the way. This first week is going to be an introduction to the exercises and program. So no worries. Now let's lace up those shoes and start moving.

Aerobic Training Exercises

Always start your aerobic activity slowly and gradually progress to your target intensity. Choose one of the following aerobic activities and do it for 10 to 15 minutes at an OMNI RPE of 1 to 2.

- Walking (outdoor or indoor)
- Biking (outdoor or indoor)
- Pool walking or exercises or swimming
- Dancing (such as salsa)
- Sports (such as tennis)

Stretching Exercises

Perform all of the following stretching exercises for 1 set of 15 seconds.

- Wrist stretch
- Neck stretches
- Hands behind back stretch
- Hands behind head stretch
- Yawn stretch
- Look over the shoulder stretch
- Calf stretch
- Hip flexor stretch
- Hamstring stretch
- Quadriceps stretch
- Inner hip stretch
- Outer hip stretch

Relaxation

Finish your exercise program by lying down and doing the slow relaxation breathing technique for 1 to 5 minutes. You can also perform Tai Chi or Qi Gong as your cool down.

One Minute Motivator:

Feeling good is not a random event.
—TM Altug, MD

166

Nutrition Diary

Keep a Food Diary

Do you find that you conveniently forget about foods eaten while standing in your kitchen making dinner or while walking past that big jar of mini candy bars on your co-worker's desk? Well, you're in good company. This is known as the "Pinocchio syndrome" (but it's a good thing our noses don't really grow with each bite or gulp we forget about).

Use your Nutrition Diary pages to record what you eat. It's a great tool to keep you aware of what you're eating and to identify what's working for you and what's not.

Suggested Menu

Let's start off with one serving of a vegetable every day. With this plan, your goal will be to vary your vegetable and fruit intake to include different color groups that provide different nutrients. For different produce options, reference the chart Color Your World on page 162.

Have one serving of vegetable from the orange group, such as 10 baby carrots. Dip in 2 tablespoons light salad dressing, if desired.

Breakfast

What I ate _____

_____

What I was doing while I ate

_____

Hunger level: **1** **2** **3** **4** **5**
Full Starving

Lunch

What I ate _____

_____

What I was doing while I ate

_____

Hunger level: **1** **2** **3** **4** **5**
Full Starving

Dinner

What I ate _____

_____

What I was doing while I ate

_____

Hunger level: **1** **2** **3** **4** **5**
Full Starving

Snack (if desired)

What I ate _____

_____

What I was doing while I ate

_____

Hunger level: **1** **2** **3** **4** **5**
Full Starving

167

the Anti-Aging Fitness
PRESCRIPTION

Activity Map

Exercise Safety Tips

• Wear appropriate exercise (proper shoes) and sports (bicycle helmet) safety gear

• Follow the 10 percent rule. Avoid increasing your program (such as walking or bicycling distance or the amount of weight lifted) more than 10 percent a week.

• Avoid doing the exact same routine two days in a row. Try to include variety and walk, swim, bike, play tennis, dance, take a yoga class or lift weights. This approach works different muscles and keeps exercise more enjoyable.

• Read exercise equipment instructions before starting.

• Don't try to keep up with another person's pace or intensity if they are at a more advanced level than you.

From Z and Tracy: Yesterday wasn't so bad, was it? Today you're going to take it easy and loosen up and stretch like your cat or dog. That's all the exercise for today.

Aerobic Training Exercises

Perform all of the following warm up exercises for 1 set of 10 reps for each exercise.

• March in place
• Shake, rattle and roll
• Trunk rotations
• Lower back cat/camel

• Heel sits with arms in front
• Heel sits with arms to side
• Hip windshield wiper

Stretching Exercises

Perform all of the following stretching exercises for 1 set of 15 seconds.

• Wrist stretch
• Neck stretches
• Hands behind back stretch
• Hands behind head stretch
• Yawn stretch
• Look over the shoulder stretch

• Calf stretch
• Hip flexor stretch
• Hamstring stretch
• Quadriceps stretch
• Inner hip stretch
• Outer hip stretch

Relaxation

Finish your exercise program by lying down and doing the slow relaxation breathing technique for 1 to 5 minutes. You can also perform Tai Chi or Qi Gong as your cool down.

Nutrition Diary

What Does a Portion Look Like?

One cup of cooked pasta, rice or potatoes: A baseball

One half cup of cooked rice: A standard-size cupcake wrapper

One serving of bread: A CD case (diameter, not thickness)

One cup of green salad: A baseball

One serving whole fruit: A tennis ball

One cup of ice cream: A baseball

Two tablespoons of peanut butter: A ping pong ball

Three ounces of cooked meat: A deck of cards

Three ounces of cooked fish: A checkbook (thickness about 3/4 inch)

Two tablespoons of salad dressing: One ice cube

Suggested Menu

Have one serving of a vegetable from the yellow/green group such as 1 cup baby spinach leaves. Have your spinach as a side salad topped with a tablespoon of light salad dressing or top a sandwich with the spinach leaves.

Breakfast

What I ate _____

_____

What I was doing while I ate

_____

Hunger level: **1**   **2**   **3**   **4**   **5**
          Full   Starving

Lunch

What I ate _____

_____

What I was doing while I ate

_____

Hunger level: **1**   **2**   **3**   **4**   **5**
          Full   Starving

Dinner

What I ate _____

_____

What I was doing while I ate

_____

Hunger level: **1**   **2**   **3**   **4**   **5**
          Full   Starving

Snack (if desired)

What I ate _____

_____

What I was doing while I ate

_____

Hunger level: **1**   **2**   **3**   **4**   **5**
          Full   Starving

169

Activity Map

Holding Your Breath with Heavy Exertion Can Be Harmful

When you are lifting weights or heavy objects, make sure you breathe out during the hardest part of the activity. Holding your breath while exerting heavy effort may rupture small blood vessels in your brain and heart and could lead to a stroke.

You should also avoid holding your breath and exerting yourself forcefully while having a bowel movement for the same reasons as above.

Athletes may use various forms of breathing but in general, you should focus on either breathing regularly during physical activity or breathing out during the hardest part of strenuous physical exertion.

From Z and Tracy: You're doing great. Now stay with us and let's do another easy and fun aerobic routine

Aerobic Training Exercises

Always start your aerobic activity slowly and gradually progress to your target intensity. Choose one of the following aerobic activities and do it for 10 to 15 minutes at an OMNI RPE of 1 to 2.

- Walking (outdoor or indoor)
- Biking (outdoor or indoor)
- Pool walking or exercises or swimming
- Dancing (such as salsa)
- Sports (such as tennis)

Stretching Exercises

Perform all of the following stretching exercises for 1 set of 15 seconds.

- Wrist stretch
- Neck stretches
- Hands behind back stretch
- Hands behind head stretch
- Yawn stretch
- Look over the shoulder stretch
- Calf stretch
- Hip flexor stretch
- Hamstring stretch
- Quadriceps stretch
- Inner hip stretch
- Outer hip stretch

Relaxation

Finish your exercise program by lying down and doing the slow relaxation breathing technique for 1 to 5 minutes. You can also perform Tai Chi or Qi Gong as your cool down.

Nutrition Diary

Simple Portion Control

For each meal, draw an imaginary line down the middle of your plate to divide it in half, and fill one half with fruit at breakfast and fruits and vegetables at lunch and dinner.

For the remaining half plate section, divide evenly between lean protein and carbohydrate-rich foods.

Suggested Menu

Have one serving of a vegetable from the green group, such as one half cup cooked broccoli florets topped with a teaspoon of toasted slivered almonds.

Breakfast

What I ate _____

_____

What I was doing while I ate

_____

Hunger level: **1   2   3   4   5**
　　　　　　Full　　　　　Starving

Lunch

What I ate _____

_____

What I was doing while I ate

_____

Hunger level: **1   2   3   4   5**
　　　　　　Full　　　　　Starving

Dinner

What I ate _____

_____

What I was doing while I ate

_____

Hunger level: **1   2   3   4   5**
　　　　　　Full　　　　　Starving

Snack (if desired)

What I ate _____

_____

What I was doing while I ate

_____

Hunger level: **1   2   3   4   5**
　　　　　　Full　　　　　Starving

171

Activity Map

F rom Z and Tracy: Let's start an easy strength training program today.

Should You Eat Before a Workout?

Some people think that working out on an empty stomach helps burn more body fat. You don't burn fat from skipping a snack or meal before a workout, and worse, you run the risk of becoming so lightheaded while working out that you can't even finish or push yourself to have an effective workout.

If you're working out after a full meal, wait about one hour after eating to get started. Otherwise, have a snack that contains mostly carbohydrate and some protein within two hours of workout. Some ideas include:

• A slice of wheat bread spread with a tablespoon of peanut butter and a tablespoon of jelly with a cup of fat-free milk.

• 8 ounces plain low fat yogurt with 1 tablespoon of raisins and 6 walnut halves.

Warm Up Exercises

Perform all of the following warm up exercises for 1 set of 10 reps for each exercise.

• March in place
• Shake, rattle and roll
• Trunk rotations
• Lower back cat/camel

• Heel sits with arms in front
• Heel sits with arms to side
• Hip windshield wiper

Strength Training Exercises

Perform all of the following muscle building and toning exercises for 1 set of 10 reps at an OMNI RPE of 1 to 2. Please go back and skim through the strength training chapter and "Before You Begin" chapter. It will help you understand how to select your weights and how to progress. Notice how we start with the largest muscles and work down to your arms and finally finish with the core exercises for the abdominals and lower back.

• Sit-to-stand squats
• Heel raises
• Partial step-ups
• Elastic pull to chest
• Elastic pull to hips
• Wingspan elastic pulls
• Dumbbell chest press

• Elastic triceps pushdown
• Dumbbell biceps curl
• Supine bridging
• Abdominal bracing
• Floor abdominal curls
• Pelvic floor contract, hold, release

Stretching Exercises

Perform all of the following stretching exercises for 1 set of 15 seconds.

• Wrist stretch
• Neck stretches
• Hands behind back stretch
• Hands behind head stretch
• Yawn stretch
• Look over the shoulder stretch

• Calf stretch
• Hip flexor stretch
• Hamstring stretch
• Quadriceps stretch
• Inner hip stretch
• Outer hip stretch

Relaxation

Finish your exercise program by lying down and doing the slow relaxation breathing technique for 1 to 5 minutes. You can also perform Tai Chi or Qi Gong as your cool down.

172

Nutrition Diary

the**Anti-Aging Fitness**
PRESCRIPTION

Tempting Treats

There's no avoiding it; unexpected food treats will tempt you along the way. For many people, work and family celebrations offer tempting treats that are difficult to pass up. Food is going to be a part of most celebrations, so it's best to face each event with a plan. Be prepared to partake in the treats at these celebrations on a limited basis. After all, your sister's Boston cream pie only rolls out once a year!

Have dessert every day, but limit your servings of high-calorie desserts or other treat such as frosted cake at a birthday celebration to once every two weeks. Some people find that they can have one high-calorie meal or "free" meal once per week (with dessert!) and still lose weight. If you have difficulty bouncing back to your healthy routine after a "free" meal, try it again once you feel more confident that you'll jump right back on your plan after your one-meal splurge.

Suggested Menu

Have one serving of a vegetable from the white/green group such as four 4-inch long stalks of celery spread with one serving of Sour Cream Spread.

Breakfast

What I ate _____

_____

What I was doing while I ate

_____

Hunger level: **1   2   3   4   5**
　　　　　　Full　　　　Starving

Lunch

What I ate _____

_____

What I was doing while I ate

_____

Hunger level: **1   2   3   4   5**
　　　　　　Full　　　　Starving

Dinner

What I ate _____

_____

What I was doing while I ate

_____

Hunger level: **1   2   3   4   5**
　　　　　　Full　　　　Starving

Snack (if desired)

What I ate _____

_____

What I was doing while I ate

_____

Hunger level: **1   2   3   4   5**
　　　　　　Full　　　　Starving

173

the **Anti-Aging Fitness**
PRESCRIPTION

Activity Map

What Is the Best Time of Day to Exercise?

Research has not identified an ideal time of day to exercise that is best for everyone. Also, keep in mind that there just isn't enough evidence for a person to do exercise in the morning on an empty stomach specifically for the purpose of burning fat as some books and magazines claim. Further research is needed in this area before making this claim. Practically speaking, "early birds" may enjoy and do well with morning exercise (or activity) while "night owls" may prefer evening exercise (or activity). So, the best time of the day to exercise is when you'll do it.

rom Z and Tracy: If your dog Sparky is starting to get some love handles, you better take him along for your activity program. While you're at it, take the TV remote away from your better half and have him or her hold Sparky's leash. Enough Three Stooges already!

Aerobic Training Exercises

Always start your aerobic activity slowly and gradually progress to your target intensity. Choose one the following aerobic activities and do it for 10 to 15 minutes.

- Walking (outdoor or indoor)
- Biking (outdoor or indoor)
- Pool walking or exercises or swimming
- Dancing (such as salsa)
- Sports (such as tennis)

Stretching Exercises

Perform all of the following stretching exercises for 1 set of 15 seconds.

- Wrist stretch
- Neck stretches
- Hands behind back stretch
- Hands behind head stretch
- Yawn stretch
- Look over the shoulder stretch
- Calf stretch
- Hip flexor stretch
- Hamstring stretch
- Quadriceps stretch
- Inner hip stretch
- Outer hip stretch

Relaxation

Finish your exercise program by lying down and doing the slow relaxation breathing technique for 1 to 5 minutes. You can also perform Tai Chi or Qi Gong as your cool down.

Anti-Aging Hint:

Most diseases are a result of some form of excess or deficiency. Correct the imbalance and you improve your health.

174

Nutrition Diary

Single-Serving Scrumptious Desserts

Take some extra time on your next trip to the grocery store to choose from the individual servings of your favorite treats. Look for frozen confections, baked treats, or salty snacks. Ideally, your treat will be: 1) 130 calories or less per serving; 2) 3 grams of saturated fat or less per serving; and 3) 1 gram of trans fat or less per serving.

Here are a few possibilities:

- Low fat ice cream sandwich
- 4 Hershey's Kisses
- Fudgesicle
- 1 ounce beef jerky
- 1 ounce bag baked chips

- Little Debbie Gingerbread Cookie or Marshmallow Treat
- 1 Hostess Light Twinkie
- A fun size piece of candy (Halloween bag candy)

The dietary guidelines call these discretionary calories. Wise wording!

Suggested Menu

Have one serving of vegetable from the red group such as one cup of low sodium tomato soup.

Breakfast

What I ate _____

_____

What I was doing while I ate

_____

Hunger level: **1   2   3   4   5**
　　　　　　　Full　　　　　Starving

Lunch

What I ate _____

_____

What I was doing while I ate

_____

Hunger level: **1   2   3   4   5**
　　　　　　　Full　　　　　Starving

Dinner

What I ate _____

_____

What I was doing while I ate

_____

Hunger level: **1   2   3   4   5**
　　　　　　　Full　　　　　Starving

Snack (if desired)

What I ate _____

_____

What I was doing while I ate

_____

Hunger level: **1   2   3   4   5**
　　　　　　　Full　　　　　Starving

175

Activity Map

Fitness For Your Mind

• Exercise: Physical activity can help prevent mental decline.

• Eat Right: Your mind and body needs adequate nutrition to keep itself healthy.

• Get Enough Sleep: Quality sleep helps improve mental health.

• Challenge Your Brain: Read a book, practice a language, play chess, work on a crossword puzzle, do math in your head, work on creative projects involving dance, music, art and writing.

For further information on keeping your brain young and fit, read Dr. Gary Small's book, *The Memory Prescription: Dr. Gary Small's 14-Day Plan to Keep Your Brain and Body Young.*

From Z and Tracy: Wasn't it Freddie Prinze from the show "Chico and the Man" who said "Loooo-king good"? Well you're really doing great for staying with us so far. For the next two days all we want you to do is loosen up, stretch and relax. See you tomorrow.

Warm Up Exercises

Perform all of the following warm up exercises for 1 set of 10 reps for each exercise.

- March in place
- Shake, rattle and roll
- Trunk rotations
- Lower back cat/camel

- Heel sits with arms in front
- Heel sits with arms to side
- Hip windshield wiper

Stretching Exercises

Perform all of the following stretching exercises for 1 set of 15 seconds.

- Wrist stretch
- Neck stretches
- Hands behind back stretch
- Hands behind head stretch
- Yawn stretch
- Look over the shoulder stretch

- Calf stretch
- Hip flexor stretch
- Hamstring stretch
- Quadriceps stretch
- Inner hip stretch
- Outer hip stretch

Relaxation

Finish your exercise program by lying down and doing the slow relaxation breathing technique for 1 to 5 minutes. You can also perform Tai Chi or Qi Gong as your cool down.

Nutrition Diary

Your Commitment

To embrace lifelong good nutrition habits, you'll need to shift your priorities to put your health first in your life. You must want to be healthy for you.

Take a few minutes to finish the thought. Some ideas, "I want to improve my health so I can take my grandchildren to the playground and play catch" or "...so I can start taking ballroom dancing lessons, something I've always wanted to do."

I want to improve my health because ...

1. _____
2. _____
3. _____

Suggested Menu

Have one serving of vegetable from the red/purple group, such as one cup cooked beets. To cook, scrub the beets but be careful not to pierce the skin, put in a microwave safe bowl with about ¼ inch of water, cover and heat for about 8 minutes. Sweet and tasty as is, no topping required.

Breakfast

What I ate _____

_____

What I was doing while I ate

_____

Hunger level: **1**   **2**   **3**   **4**   **5**
         Full   Starving

Lunch

What I ate _____

_____

What I was doing while I ate

_____

Hunger level: **1**   **2**   **3**   **4**   **5**
         Full   Starving

Dinner

What I ate _____

_____

What I was doing while I ate

_____

Hunger level: **1**   **2**   **3**   **4**   **5**
         Full   Starving

Snack (if desired)

What I ate _____

_____

What I was doing while I ate

_____

Hunger level: **1**   **2**   **3**   **4**   **5**
         Full   Starving

the Anti-Aging Fitness PRESCRIPTION

Activity Map

Fashion Sense

Pamela Burns, a fashion consultant in the Washington DC area offers some clothing selection SOS:

• Weed out your closet. Outdated trendy-colored clothing must go.

• Choose one new piece and keep the rest classic. An updated shoe can bring your outfit from so-last-year to just right. Always-in-style colors include white, black, gray and navy.

• Women should keep sweater sets with a jewel neckline, basic blouses in small feminine flowery prints, basic polo shirts, oxford shirts, turtlenecks and straight skirts that hit at the knee.

• For men, flat-front pants are a good choice but if they are a difficult fit (a little too much girth in the mid section) look for one-pleat pants.

Your Bodyweight:_____

From Z and Tracy: Congratulations, you just finished the first phase of your program. Doesn't it feel good to do something that's fun and easy? Next week we move up the intensity a little. Hang in there. We'll chat again tomorrow.

Warm Up Exercises

Perform all of the following warm up exercises for 1 set of 10 reps for each exercise.

• March in place
• Shake, rattle and roll
• Trunk rotations
• Lower back cat / camel

• Heel sits with arms in front
• Heel sits with arms to side
• Hip windshield wiper

Stretching Exercises

Perform all of the following stretching exercises for 1 set of 15 seconds.

• Wrist stretch
• Neck stretches
• Hands behind back stretch
• Hands behind head stretch
• Yawn stretch
• Look over the shoulder stretch

• Calf stretch
• Hip flexor stretch
• Hamstring stretch
• Quadriceps stretch
• Inner hip stretch
• Outer hip stretch

Relaxation

Finish your exercise program by lying down and doing the slow relaxation breathing technique for 1 to 5 minutes. You can also perform Tai Chi or Qi Gong as your cool down.

Did You Know That...

One pound of lean body mass (muscle) burns 14 calories per day and 1 pound of fat burns 2 calories per day. So build more muscle and burn more calories at rest!

178

Nutrition Diary

Steps to Good Health

Shoot for simple, gradual changes in your eating habits that you can follow for the rest of your life. Write down only what you know you can achieve, and you'll have a chance to set loftier goals as you make progress. If you're not a regular exerciser, you might try, "Once a day, I will get up from my desk and walk for 10 minutes without stopping," and if you need to up your intake of vegetables, you might say, "At lunch I'll choose 1 cup of raw vegetables from the salad bar to go with my meal."

I plan to follow these steps to better health ...

1. _____

2. _____

3. _____

Suggested Menu

Have one serving of a vegetable from the yellow/green group such as a medium size ear of yellow corn on the cob. If corn isn't in season, try two small frozen cobs of corn, the next best thing to fresh picked.

Breakfast

What I ate _____

_____

What I was doing while I ate

_____

Hunger level: **1**   **2**   **3**   **4**   **5**
          Full   Starving

Lunch

What I ate _____

_____

What I was doing while I ate

_____

Hunger level: **1**   **2**   **3**   **4**   **5**
          Full   Starving

Dinner

What I ate _____

_____

What I was doing while I ate

_____

Hunger level: **1**   **2**   **3**   **4**   **5**
          Full   Starving

Snack (if desired)

What I ate _____

_____

What I was doing while I ate

_____

Hunger level: **1**   **2**   **3**   **4**   **5**
          Full   Starving

One Minute Motivator:

Well begun is half done.
—Aristotle

the **Anti-Aging Fitness**
PRESCRIPTION

Activity Map

The Tortoise Beats The Hare

You've probably heard of the children's fable about how a slow but steady turtle beats the speedy hare. There are many lessons we could take away from this simple story. One could be that so many people speed through life and never really enjoy ride. The second could be that life really doesn't have a finish line where the first one there wins a prize. The third might be that slow and steady gets the job done without unnecessary stress.

So try to take the slower but scenic route through life as much as you can.

From Z and Tracy: We hope you had a good day yesterday. This week you will enter Phase 2 which focuses on building your body, mind and improving your eating habits. This week we'll be increasing the length of your aerobic workout by 5 minutes and you can also pick up the pace a little.

Aerobic Training Exercises

Always start your aerobic activity slowly and gradually progress to your target intensity. Choose one the following aerobic activities and do it for 15 to 20 minutes at an OMNI RPE of 2 to 3.

- Walking (outdoor or indoor)
- Biking (outdoor or indoor)
- Pool walking or exercises or swimming
- Dancing (such as salsa)
- Sports (such as tennis)

Stretching Exercises

Perform all of the following stretching exercises for 1 set of 15 seconds.

- Wrist stretch
- Neck stretches
- Hands behind back stretch
- Hands behind head stretch
- Yawn stretch
- Look over the shoulder stretch
- Calf stretch
- Hip flexor stretch
- Hamstring stretch
- Quadriceps stretch
- Inner hip stretch
- Outer hip stretch

180

Nutrition Diary

The Six Classes of Nutrients

Protein
- Builds and repairs body tissue
- Major component of enzymes, hormones, and antibodies

Carbohydrate
- Provides a major source of fuel
- Supplies dietary fiber

Fats
- Chief storage form of energy
- Insulates and protects vital organs
- Aids absorption of fat-soluble vitamins

Vitamins
- Help promote and regulate various chemical reactions and bodily processes
- Help release energy from food

Minerals
- Enable enzymes to function
- A component of hormones

Water
- Enables chemical reactions to occur
- Essential for life

Suggested Menu

Now that you're getting used to having a vegetable serving every day, let's add a fruit serving too. Also, starting today, begin tracking your fruit and vegetable intake.

Have one serving of vegetable from the orange group such as one small sliced yellow squash (try dipping it in three tablespoons light salad dressing) and one serving of fruit from the red/purple group, such as 1 cup fresh or frozen (unsweetened) strawberries.

Breakfast

What I ate _____

_____

What I was doing while I ate

_____

Hunger level: **1**   **2**   **3**   **4**   **5**
  Full   Starving

Lunch

What I ate _____

_____

What I was doing while I ate

_____

Hunger level: **1**   **2**   **3**   **4**   **5**
  Full   Starving

Dinner

What I ate _____

_____

What I was doing while I ate

_____

Hunger level: **1**   **2**   **3**   **4**   **5**
  Full   Starving

Snack (if desired)

What I ate _____

_____

What I was doing while I ate

_____

Hunger level: **1**   **2**   **3**   **4**   **5**
  Full   Starving

181

the Anti-Aging Fitness
PRESCRIPTION

Activity Map

You Can't Choose Where You Lose

You can't choose where you lose fat from a particular area of the body. If that were true, then chewing gum would give you a thin face. To examine this point, a study had subjects perform 5,004 conventional hook lying sit-ups over a 27-day period. Their results revealed that sit-ups did not preferentially reduce abdominal fat cells. Unless you want to repeat their study, we suggest you stick with the basics of healthy eating and sensible exercise.

From Z and Tracy: Today we've added a few more reps to your strength program and included two new, fun balance exercises. Also you'll be doing two strength workouts this week. We'll check up with you in a few days. Don't worry, both of us will be watching over you to make sure you're okay.

Warm Up Exercises

Perform all of the following warm up exercises for 1 set of 10 reps for each exercise.

- March in place
- Shake, rattle and roll
- Trunk rotations
- Lower back cat/camel
- Heel sits with arms in front
- Heel sits with arms to side
- Hip windshield wiper

Strength Training Exercises

Perform all of the following muscle building and toning exercises for 1 set of 15 reps at an OMNI RPE of 2 to 3.

- Sit-to-stand squats
- Heel raises
- Partial step-ups
- Elastic pull to chest
- Elastic pull to hips
- Wingspan elastic pulls
- Dumbbell chest press
- Elastic triceps pushdown
- Dumbbell biceps curl
- Supine bridging
- Abdominal bracing
- Floor abdominal curls
- Pelvic floor contract, hold, release

Balance Exercises

Perform both balance exercises for 2 sets of 15 seconds.

- Very slow motion balancing and walking in place
- Dancer's balance

Stretching Exercises

Perform all of the following stretching exercises for 1 set of 15 seconds.

- Wrist stretch
- Neck stretches
- Hands behind back stretch
- Hands behind head stretch
- Yawn stretch
- Look over the shoulder stretch
- Calf stretch
- Hip flexor stretch
- Hamstring stretch
- Quadriceps stretch
- Inner hip stretch
- Outer hip stretch

Relaxation Exercises

Finish your exercise program by lying down and doing the slow relaxation breathing technique for 1 to 5 minutes. You can also per-form Tai Chi or Qi Gong as your cool down.

Nutrition Diary

Building Blocks for your Body

Walk into a gym anywhere and you'll find weight lifters extolling the benefits of a high protein diet. Protein powders, steak and tuna are the staples for body builders across the land. Here's the skinny on protein: after a workout, your muscle needs a little bit of protein for muscle repair. Your enzymes, hormones and antibodies are made mostly from protein. But it's your glycogen stores and the carbohydrate in your diet that are the catalyst to push yourself during either a strength training workout or an aerobic workout.

See the Mix 'n Match Anti-Aging Meal Plan on page 160 for the right amount of lean mean proteins to add to your day.

Suggested Menu

Have one serving of fruit from the yellow/green group such as 2 sliced kiwi and one serving of vegetable from the yellow/green group such as one sliced yellow pepper. Dip in 2 tablespoons light salad dressing.

Breakfast

What I ate _____

_____

What I was doing while I ate

_____

Hunger level: **1**   **2**   **3**   **4**   **5**
Full   Starving

Lunch

What I ate _____

_____

What I was doing while I ate

_____

Hunger level: **1**   **2**   **3**   **4**   **5**
Full   Starving

Dinner

What I ate _____

_____

What I was doing while I ate

_____

Hunger level: **1**   **2**   **3**   **4**   **5**
Full   Starving

Snack (if desired)

What I ate _____

_____

What I was doing while I ate

_____

Hunger level: **1**   **2**   **3**   **4**   **5**
Full   Starving

183

the**Anti-Aging Fitness**
PRESCRIPTION

Activity Map

Improving Recovery Between Workouts

• Try some gentle Yoga, Tai Chi, or Qi Gong.

• Try stretching in a pool to loosen stiff muscles.

• Drink up! Replenish body fluids and electrolytes by drinking water, fruit and vegetable juices and other caffeine-free beverages.

• Take up a hobby such as sculpting, painting, playing music and make time for reading, traveling and learning to ensure you have a well-rounded social life which can help prevent mental burnout.

• Use passive rest techniques such as sleep, massage, warm shower, listening to relaxing music, and diaphragmatic breathing.

Aerobic Training Exercises

Always start your aerobic activity slowly and gradually progress to your target intensity. Choose one the following aerobic activities and do it for 15 to 20 minutes at an OMNI RPE of 2 to 3.

• Walking (outdoor or indoor)
• Biking (outdoor or indoor)
• Pool walking or exercises or swimming
• Dancing (such as salsa)

• Sports (such as tennis)

Stretching Exercises

Perform all of the following stretching exercises for 1 set of 15 seconds.

• Wrist stretch
• Neck stretches
• Hands behind back stretch
• Hands behind head stretch
• Yawn stretch
• Look over the shoulder stretch

• Calf stretch
• Hip flexor stretch
• Hamstring stretch
• Quadriceps stretch
• Inner hip stretch
• Outer hip stretch

Relaxation

Finish your exercise program by lying down and doing the slow relaxation breathing technique for 1 to 5 minutes. You can also perform Tai Chi or Qi Gong as your cool down.

184

Nutrition Diary

Carbohydrate Confusion

Carbohydrate-rich foods are your body's preferred source of blood glucose for brain function. Simply put, your central nervous system and brain depend on a continual supply of glucose. So what happens when you eliminate the bulk of carbohydrate-rich foods from your diet? Your body turns to liver glycogen stores to maintain blood glucose, then gluconeogenesis, or making glucose from protein, kicks in. This can take a little while, so you may lose energy if you're exercising.

Avid followers of low-carbohydrate diets, around 10 to 60 grams a day, often choose few and unvaried choices of fruits and vegetables (on many of the plans fruits and vegetables are classified as good or bad) and they're the whole crux of the anti-aging eating plan. So keep the fruits and vegetables coming!

Suggested Menu

Have one serving of fruit from the orange group such as 5 dried apricot halves and one serving of vegetable from the white/green group such 8 spears cooked asparagus, topping suggestion: 1 teaspoon olive oil, ¼ teaspoon no-salt seasoning and lemon juice

Breakfast

What I ate _____

_____

What I was doing while I ate

_____

Hunger level: **1**   **2**   **3**   **4**   **5**
          Full   Starving

Lunch

What I ate _____

_____

What I was doing while I ate

_____

Hunger level: **1**   **2**   **3**   **4**   **5**
          Full   Starving

Dinner

What I ate _____

_____

What I was doing while I ate

_____

Hunger level: **1**   **2**   **3**   **4**   **5**
          Full   Starving

Snack (if desired)

What I ate _____

_____

What I was doing while I ate

_____

Hunger level: **1**   **2**   **3**   **4**   **5**
          Full   Starving

Activity Map

Lift It Right to Prevent Back Injury

• Plan your lift. Determine how you are going to hold the object and where you are going to move it.

• Lift the object smoothly and avoid jerky motions.

• When lifting an object, plant your feet firmly on the ground.

• When lifting an object, bend at the knees, not the back.

• Keep lifted objects close to the body.

• Don't twist when lifting or carrying objects. (A simple rule to remember: your nose should follow your toes).

• Before you lift something heavy tense your abdominals. A simple rule to remember is "lock and load."

Warm Up Exercises

Perform all of the following warm up exercises for 1 set of 10 reps for each exercise.

• March in place
• Shake, rattle and roll
• Trunk rotations
• Lower back cat / camel

• Heel sits with arms in front
• Heel sits with arms to side
• Hip windshield wiper

Stretching Exercises

Perform all of the following stretching exercises for 1 set of 15 seconds.

• Wrist stretch
• Neck stretches
• Hands behind back stretch
• Hands behind head stretch
• Yawn stretch
• Look over the shoulder stretch

• Calf stretch
• Hip flexor stretch
• Hamstring stretch
• Quadriceps stretch
• Inner hip stretch
• Outer hip stretch

Relaxation

Finish your exercise program by lying down and doing the slow relaxation breathing technique for 1 to 5 minutes. You can also perform Tai Chi or Qi Gong as your cool down.

Nutrition Diary

Whole Grain Wisdom

With dozens of options of bread, crackers and cereals, it's hard to choose. Fiber helps prevent constipation, can help manage blood sugar for diabetics, may cut the risk of heart disease, diverticulosis and cancer. Here are some guidelines on finding whole grain products.

• Look for breads and cereals that are whole grain and are high in fiber.

• Choose breads and crackers that list whole grains on the ingredients list and have at leave 2 grams of fiber per serving.

• Avoid high-sugar cereals. The sugar replaces too much of the fiber even if the cereal is whole grain.

• Use the "5" rule, the food should have less than 5 grams of sugar and at least 5 grams of fiber in a serving.

Suggested Menu

Have one serving of vegetable from the red/purple group and one serving of fruit from the white/green group. Make a dish with one pear and one cup red cabbage. Coat a skillet with cooking spray, add 1 teaspoon canola oil and heat over medium heat. Stir fry 2 tablespoons chopped white onion until translucent, add 1 finely chopped pear with the skin on, stir fry for 2 minutes, add 1 cup fresh shredded cabbage and heat for 7 minutes. Turn down heat to low, then add 1 teaspoon brown sugar and 1 teaspoon red wine vinegar and heat for another 5 minutes.

Breakfast

What I ate _____

_____

What I was doing while I ate

_____

Hunger level: **1**   **2**   **3**   **4**   **5**
              Full   Starving

Lunch

What I ate _____

_____

What I was doing while I ate

_____

Hunger level: **1**   **2**   **3**   **4**   **5**
              Full   Starving

Dinner

What I ate _____

_____

What I was doing while I ate

_____

Hunger level: **1**   **2**   **3**   **4**   **5**
              Full   Starving

Snack (if desired)

What I ate _____

_____

What I was doing while I ate

_____

Hunger level: **1**   **2**   **3**   **4**   **5**
              Full   Starving

187

the **Anti-Aging Fitness**
PRESCRIPTION

Activity Map

Lifting Belts: To Use Or Not To Use

The appropriateness of wearing a lifting belt depends on the type of exercise and the amount of weight you will be lifting. Some experts recommend using weightlifting belts only for exercises that place major stress on the lower back and involve near maximum or maximum loads (such as heavy barbell squats and deadlifts). Training with a weightlifting belt is not enough to prevent injury. To help prevent injury, you need to adhere to proper form and follow sound training strategies.

Warm Up Exercises

Perform all of the following warm up exercises for 1 set of 10 reps for each exercise.

- March in place
- Shake, rattle and roll
- Trunk rotations
- Lower back cat / camel
- Heel sits with arms in front
- Heel sits with arms to side
- Hip windshield wiper

Strength Training Exercises

Perform all of the following muscle building and toning exercises for 1 set of 15 reps at an OMNI RPE of 2 to 3.

- Sit-to-stand squats
- Heel raises
- Partial step-ups
- Elastic pull to chest
- Elastic pull to hips
- Wingspan elastic pulls
- Dumbbell chest press
- Elastic triceps pushdown
- Dumbbell biceps curl
- Supine bridging
- Abdominal bracing
- Floor abdominal curls
- Pelvic floor contract, hold, release

Balance Exercises

Perform both balance exercises for 2 sets of 15 seconds.

- Very slow motion balancing and walking in place
- Dancer's balance

Stretching Exercises

Perform all of the following stretching exercises for 1 set of 15 seconds.

- Wrist stretch
- Neck stretches
- Hands behind back stretch
- Hands behind head stretch
- Yawn stretch
- Look over the shoulder stretch
- Calf stretch
- Hip flexor stretch
- Hamstring stretch
- Quadriceps stretch
- Inner hip stretch
- Outer hip stretch

Relaxation

Finish your exercise program by lying down and doing the slow relaxation breathing technique for 1 to 5 minutes. You can also perform Tai Chi or Qi Gong as your cool down.

188

Nutrition Diary

Fat Facts

Saturated fat: Foods rich in saturated fat include butter, meats, animal fats, tropical oils and full-fat dairy products. These fats can raise LDL blood levels (low density lipoprotein).

Unsaturated fat: These fats help maintain good HDL blood levels (high density lipoprotein). These include vegetable oils, seeds, nuts and avocados.

Hydrogenated or trans fatty acids: Baked goods, cookies, crackers, candy and margarine have the most trans fats. These fats not only raise LDL levels, but they can lower healthy HDL levels, making them more dangerous than saturated fats. Many foods may boast "trans-free" on the package front. You may have been told to check the product ingredients for the words "partially hydrogenated oil" but unfortunately this is not going to tell you how much trans fat is in the food. Check with the manufacturer for exact nutrition facts.

Suggested Menu

Have one serving of fruit from the red group such as one half pink grapefruit and one serving of vegetable from the green group such as one cup cooked kale, top with 1 teaspoon olive oil and ¼ teaspoon no-salt seasoning.

Breakfast

What I ate _____

_____

What I was doing while I ate

_____

Hunger level: **1**   **2**   **3**   **4**   **5**
　　　　　　Full　　　　　Starving

Lunch

What I ate _____

_____

What I was doing while I ate

_____

Hunger level: **1**   **2**   **3**   **4**   **5**
　　　　　　Full　　　　　Starving

Dinner

What I ate _____

_____

What I was doing while I ate

_____

Hunger level: **1**   **2**   **3**   **4**   **5**
　　　　　　Full　　　　　Starving

Snack (if desired)

What I ate _____

_____

What I was doing while I ate

_____

Hunger level: **1**   **2**   **3**   **4**   **5**
　　　　　　Full　　　　　Starving

189

Activity Map

Abdominal Mania

Are your abdominals the most important muscle in your body? You might get that impression if you watch all the TV commercials promoting abdominal exercise machines. Most people do abdominal exercise to try and get rid of the fat around their middle. The truth is that the fat around your waist is primarily as a result of poor nutrition and lifestyle habits.

So in the end, it really comes down to what is in your refrigerator, what you put on your plate, and what you fill your glass with that is going to help you get that toned midsection.

Aerobic Training Exercises

Always start your aerobic activity slowly and gradually progress to your target intensity. Choose one the following aerobic activities and do it for 15 to 20 minutes at an OMNI RPE of 2 to 3.

- Walking (outdoor or indoor)
- Biking (outdoor or indoor)
- Pool walking or exercises or swimming
- Dancing (such as salsa)
- Sports (such as tennis)

Stretching Exercises

Perform all of the following stretching exercises for 1 set of 15 seconds.

- Wrist stretch
- Neck stretches
- Hands behind back stretch
- Hands behind head stretch
- Yawn stretch
- Look over the shoulder stretch
- Calf stretch
- Hip flexor stretch
- Hamstring stretch
- Quadriceps stretch
- Inner hip stretch
- Outer hip stretch

Relaxation

Finish your exercise program by lying down and doing the slow relaxation breathing technique for 1 to 5 minutes. You can also perform Tai Chi or Qi Gong as your cool down.

Nutrition Diary

Tricky Trans Fats

With the new labeling requirements for listing trans fats on the nutrition facts label, don't be fooled into believing that trans-free automatically means healthy. Fats lend a certain mouth feel to foods, a particular crispiness to crackers and cookies and creaminess to candies, margarine and other treats. It's hard for the manufacturer to eliminate the trans fats and maintain this crispiness and creaminess, but it's not impossible. You may find that the manufacturer has replaced trans fats with something else that may be just as unhealthy. Steer clear of ingredients high in saturated fat such as palm or coconut oil (tropical oils) or stearic-acid rich vegetable oil sometimes listed as interesterified vegetable oil, a saturated fat that doesn't appear to raise, nor does it lower your blood cholesterol level. So check your label before deeming your trans-free food as healthy.

Suggested Menu

Have one serving of fruit and vegetable from the orange group, such as one orange and one serving of vegetable from the orange group, such as one cup butternut squash soup (available boxed or in a can).

Breakfast

What I ate _____

_____

What I was doing while I ate

_____

Hunger level: **1**   **2**   **3**   **4**   **5**
         Full   Starving

Lunch

What I ate _____

_____

What I was doing while I ate

_____

Hunger level: **1**   **2**   **3**   **4**   **5**
         Full   Starving

Dinner

What I ate _____

_____

What I was doing while I ate

_____

Hunger level: **1**   **2**   **3**   **4**   **5**
         Full   Starving

Snack (if desired)

What I ate _____

_____

What I was doing while I ate

_____

Hunger level: **1**   **2**   **3**   **4**   **5**
         Full   Starving

191

the **Anti-Aging Fitness**
PRESCRIPTION

Activity Map

Cellulite Wars

Cellulite — you try to brush it off, roll it off, rub it off, steam it off, dissolve it off, and use "special" machines to exercise it off.

Cellulite is not a true medical condition but a non-technical term for the deposits of fat under the skin.

You can reduce the appearance of cellulite by eating a balanced diet to avoid excess calories and thus, prevent becoming overweight.

Second, you should engage in a strength and flexibility training program to promote good muscle tone.

Third, engage in an aerobic program (for example, walking, biking, or swimming) in order to help burn calories and prevent weight gain.

Your Bodyweight:_____

From Z and Tracy: You have two solid weeks of exercise and healthy eating under your belt (so to speak). Do you find that you're smiling a little more often? Ask your family or coworkers and they'll tell you how much better you look. Go do something fun today and we'll catch up with you tomorrow.

Warm Up Exercises

Perform all of the following warm up exercises for 1 set of 10 reps for each exercise.

- March in place
- Shake, rattle and roll
- Trunk rotations
- Lower back cat / camel
- Heel sits with arms in front
- Heel sits with arms to side
- Hip windshield wiper

Stretching Exercises

Perform all of the following stretching exercises for 1 set of 15 seconds.

- Wrist stretch
- Neck stretches
- Hands behind back stretch
- Hands behind head stretch
- Yawn stretch
- Look over the shoulder stretch
- Calf stretch
- Hip flexor stretch
- Hamstring stretch
- Quadriceps stretch
- Inner hip stretch
- Outer hip stretch

Relaxation

Finish your exercise program by lying down and doing the slow relaxation breathing technique for 1 to 5 minutes. You can also perform Tai Chi or Qi Gong as your cool down.

Did You Know That...

There are approximately 206 bones in the human body, which includes 33 vertebrae in the spine, and 12 pairs of ribs. Exercise helps keep all these bones strong.

Nutrition Diary

Your Reward System

A little self-praise in the form of a reward can work wonders to keep you on track with your new lifestyle. The reward you choose should be something above and beyond your normal routine.

Be mindful of what this reward represents. What challenges did you overcome to keep on track with your exercise and eating plan? Remember the time you exercised when you didn't feel like moving a muscle or the time you pushed away from the table when you normally would have kept eating.

Circle the rewards that appeal to you. Use them every two weeks (we'll remind you) to celebrate your dedication to your program.

A relaxing bath

A massage or facial

A manicure or haircut

A book or CD

A visit to a friend

A day trip

Lessons for an activity you've always wanted to try

New workout shoes, clothes, or equipment

Tickets to a sporting event

A new household tool or gadget

Suggested Menu

Have one serving of fruit from the red group such as 1½ cups cubed watermelon and one serving of vegetable from the yellow/green group such as ½ cup cooked peas, serving suggestion: 1 teaspoon trans-free margarine and a sprinkle of no-salt seasoning.

Breakfast

What I ate _____

_____

What I was doing while I ate

_____

Hunger level: **1**   **2**   **3**   **4**   **5**
               Full   Starving

Lunch

What I ate _____

_____

What I was doing while I ate

_____

Hunger level: **1**   **2**   **3**   **4**   **5**
               Full   Starving

Dinner

What I ate _____

_____

What I was doing while I ate

_____

Hunger level: **1**   **2**   **3**   **4**   **5**
               Full   Starving

Snack (if desired)

What I ate _____

_____

What I was doing while I ate

_____

Hunger level: **1**   **2**   **3**   **4**   **5**
               Full   Starving

193

the Anti-Aging Fitness
PRESCRIPTION

Activity Map

Quitting Smoking And Weight Gain

Some people who stop smoking gain weight. The good news is that quitting smoking significantly improves your health and decreases many health related risk factors. Some studies have found exercise to be beneficial for delaying weight gain after quitting smoking. In addition to exercise, you should also avoid food as a substitute for cigarettes, and establish a support group (family, friends).

From Z and Tracy: Okay now we enter week three and we're adding another 5 minutes to your aerobic workout. Also this week you'll be doing 4 aerobic workouts. It'll be easy, you'll see.

Aerobic Training Exercises

Always start your aerobic activity slowly and gradually progress to your target intensity. Choose one the following aerobic activities and do it for 20 to 25 minutes at an OMNI RPE of 3 to 4.

- Walking (outdoor or indoor)
- Biking (outdoor or indoor)
- Pool walking or exercises or swimming
- Dancing (such as salsa)
- Sports (such as tennis)

Stretching Exercises

Perform all of the following stretching exercises for 1 set of 15 to 30 seconds.

- Wrist stretch
- Neck stretches
- Hands behind back stretch
- Hands behind head stretch
- Yawn stretch
- Look over the shoulder stretch
- Calf stretch
- Hip flexor stretch
- Hamstring stretch
- Quadriceps stretch
- Inner hip stretch
- Outer hip stretch

Relaxation

Finish your exercise program by lying down and doing the slow relaxation breathing technique for 1 to 5 minutes. You can also perform Tai Chi or Qi Gong as your cool down.

Nutrition Diary

Vitamins and Minerals

Vitamins and minerals serve many purposes in our bodies, and they ARE essential to our well being. When you increase your intake of fruits and vegetables and calcium-rich foods, as you do very nicely with the anti-aging plan, you get nearly everything you need from your foods and drink. But what do vitamins and minerals actually do in our body?

Vitamins help promote and regulate various chemical reactions and body processes. They participate in reactions to release energy from food.

Minerals are critical for enabling enzymes to function properly in the chemical reactions that happen in your body. They're also a component of hormones and an essential part of bone and nerve impulses.

Breakfast

What I ate _____

_____

What I was doing while I ate

_____

Hunger level: **1**   **2**   **3**   **4**   **5**
      Full   Starving

Lunch

What I ate _____

_____

What I was doing while I ate

_____

Hunger level: **1**   **2**   **3**   **4**   **5**
      Full   Starving

Dinner

What I ate _____

_____

What I was doing while I ate

_____

Hunger level: **1**   **2**   **3**   **4**   **5**
      Full   Starving

Snack (if desired)

What I ate _____

_____

What I was doing while I ate

_____

Hunger level: **1**   **2**   **3**   **4**   **5**
      Full   Starving

Suggested Menu

Starting this week, let's add a serving of calcium-rich foods to the day. Have one cup fat-free milk. Have one serving of fruit from the red/purple group such as one cup fresh or frozen, unsweetened raspberries and one serving of vegetable from the red group such as one small fresh sliced tomato. Try topping your sandwich with the tomato.

195

Activity Map

Stress And Weight Gain

Chronic stress can trigger a series of reactions in the body and could cause fat retention by select cells. The key is to figure out the specific stressors in your life and learn to minimize and control them. Stress can lead to eating disorders. Keep in mind that an overemphasis on thinness can also be an unnecessary stressor in life and thus contribute to the weight gain.

The way a person handles stress appears to be more important than the actual stress itself. For instance, one person may perceive a particular situation as a stressful event and another person may perceive it as a challenge to rise to the occasion. So what floats your boat may sink your neighbor's ship.

196

From Z and Tracy: Today we are increasing your strength program to 1 to 2 sets of 10 to 15 reps and increasing your balance to 1 set of 30 seconds. See you in a few days.

Warm Up Exercisesk

Perform all of the following warm up exercises for 1 set of 10 reps for each exercise.

- March in place
- Shake, rattle and roll
- Trunk rotations
- Lower back cat / camel
- Heel sits with arms in front
- Heel sits with arms to side
- Hip windshield wiper

Stretching Exercises

Perform all of the following muscle building and toning exercises for 1 to 2 sets of 10 to 15 reps at an OMNI RPE of 3 to 4.

- Wall ball squats
- Heel raises
- Partial step-ups
- Elastic pull to chest
- Elastic pull to hips
- Wingspan elastic pulls
- Dumbbell chest press
- Elastic triceps push-down
- Dumbbell biceps curl
- Supine bridging
- Abdominal bracing
- Floor abdominal curls
- Pelvic floor contract, hold, release

Balance Exercises

Perform both balance exercises for 1 set of 30 seconds.

- Very slow motion balancing and walking in place
- Dancer's balance

Stretching Exercises

Perform all of the following stretching exercises for 1 set of 15 to 30 seconds.

- Wrist stretch
- Neck stretches
- Hands behind back stretch
- Hands behind head stretch
- Yawn stretch
- Look over the shoulder stretch
- Calf stretch
- Hip flexor stretch
- Hamstring stretch
- Quadriceps stretch
- Inner hip stretch
- Outer hip stretch

Relaxation

Finish your exercise program by lying down and doing the slow relaxation breathing technique for 1 to 5 minutes. You can also perform Tai Chi or Qi Gong as your cool down.

Nutrition Diary

Water Water Everywhere

Water is absolutely essential for life. You can't store it or conserve it. But what function does water provide for us? The H2O in your body enables chemical reactions to occur. This is why doctors get so concerned about dehydration; your metabolism slows considerably when your body is running low on water. Also, when you get overheated from exercise or from a hot environment, water is essential for cooling your body. Perspiration is your body's cooling mechanism; the water leaves your pores, and as it evaporates there is a cooling effect on your skin. When your water stores run too low, perspiration slows and you can't cool down effectively. Water also lubricates our joints and helps speed along the digestive process.

Your new anti-aging diet will boost your water intake from all the fruits and vegetables. But shoot for 64 ounces of fluids every day.

Suggested Menu

Have one serving of fruit from the yellow/green group such as two kiwi and one serving of vegetable from the green group such as ½ cup cooked kale, serving suggestion: top with ½ teaspoon no-salt seasoning and 1 teaspoon olive oil.

Have one serving Peanutty Ricotta Spread as your calcium-rich food. This keeps for up to 6 days in the refrigerator or up to 30 days in the freezer. Serving suggestion: dip 6 graham cracker squares in the spread.

Breakfast

What I ate _____

_____

What I was doing while I ate

_____

Hunger level: **1**   **2**   **3**   **4**   **5**
       Full   Starving

Lunch

What I ate _____

_____

What I was doing while I ate

_____

Hunger level: **1**   **2**   **3**   **4**   **5**
       Full   Starving

Dinner

What I ate _____

_____

What I was doing while I ate

_____

Hunger level: **1**   **2**   **3**   **4**   **5**
       Full   Starving

Snack (if desired)

What I ate _____

_____

What I was doing while I ate

_____

Hunger level: **1**   **2**   **3**   **4**   **5**
       Full   Starving

197

the Anti-Aging Fitness
PRESCRIPTION

Activity Map

Massage Your Stress Away

Massage can have many beneficial aspects such as reducing muscle tension, increasing a sense of well being, helping to control stress and anxiety and helping to decrease pain. Include massage into your day.

• Learn simple massage techniques and trade off doing massages with your partner.

• Hire a professional massage therapist.

• Use a shower massager.

• Get a chair massager for your home.

• Use simple hand-held massage devices such as a rope massager, massager roller, or massage cane.

Aerobic Training Exercises

Always start your aerobic activity slowly and gradually progress to your target intensity. Choose one the following aerobic activities and do it for 20 to 25 minutes at an OMNI RPE of 3 to 4.

• Walking (outdoor or indoor)
• Biking (outdoor or indoor)
• Pool walking or exercises or swimming
• Dancing (such as salsa)
• Sports (such as tennis)

Stretching Exercises

Perform all of the following stretching exercises for 1 set of 15 to 30 seconds.

• Wrist stretch
• Neck stretches
• Hands behind back stretch
• Hands behind head stretch
• Yawn stretch
• Look over the shoulder stretch
• Calf stretch
• Hip flexor stretch
• Hamstring stretch
• Quadriceps stretch
• Inner hip stretch
• Outer hip stretch

Relaxation

Finish your exercise program by lying down and doing the slow relaxation breathing technique for 1 to 5 minutes. You can also perform Tai Chi or Qi Gong as your cool down.

Nutrition Diary

What to Drink

Drinks can go down easy. Beverages such as soda, hot chocolate, specialty coffee shop drinks, lemonade, sweetened iced tea, juice, alcohol and milkshakes can pile on the calories with very little effort. All of these drinks would count as discretionary calories according to the 2005 food guide pyramid. Wouldn't you rather save up for your 130-calorie treat every day?

Drinking rarely takes the place of eating. High-calorie drinks can put you over the top calorie-wise for the day. Our minds don't register satiety from drinking, so be mindful of calorie-rich beverages. And keep plain water, flavored seltzer, tea and other very low or non-caloric beverages in your day.

Suggested Menu

Have one serving of fruit from the orange/yellow fruit such as two tangelos (serve topped with1 cup low fat fruit-flavored yogurt), and one serving of vegetable from the red/purple group such as 1 cup of red cabbage, serving suggestion, make a salad with 1 cup romaine lettuce and 1 cup shredded red cabbage, make it a meal with 3 ounces of sliced, roasted chicken, 1 tablespoon of peanuts and 2 tablespoons of an Asian sesame salad dressing.

Breakfast

What I ate _____

_____

What I was doing while I ate

_____

Hunger level: **1** **2** **3** **4** **5**
Full Starving

Lunch

What I ate _____

_____

What I was doing while I ate

_____

Hunger level: **1** **2** **3** **4** **5**
Full Starving

Dinner

What I ate _____

_____

What I was doing while I ate

_____

Hunger level: **1** **2** **3** **4** **5**
Full Starving

Snack (if desired)

What I ate _____

_____

What I was doing while I ate

_____

Hunger level: **1** **2** **3** **4** **5**
Full Starving

199

the**Anti-Aging Fitness**
PRESCRIPTION

Activity Map

Natural Pain Relief Strategies

If you have general muscle and joint aches then the following strategies may help you reduce your discomfort.

• Get medical help: See your healthcare provider and learn how to protect your joints, how to conserve your energy, how to perform daily activities with painfree postures and how to lift items with good technique to prevent pain.

• Use mind/body movements: Try Tai Chi, Qi Gong, or yoga.

• Get a massage or try acupuncture.

One Minute Motivator:

If we could give every individual the right amount of nourishment and exercise, not too little and not too much, we would have found the safest way to health.
—Hippocrates

Aerobic Training Exercises

Always start your aerobic activity slowly and gradually progress to your target intensity. Choose one the following aerobic activities and do it for 20 to 25 minutes at an OMNI RPE of 3 to 4.

• Walking (outdoor or indoor)
• Biking (outdoor or indoor)
• Pool walking or exercises or swimming
• Dancing (such as salsa)
• Sports (such as tennis)

Stretching Exercises

Perform all of the following stretching exercises for 1 set of 15 to 30 seconds.

• Wrist stretch
• Neck stretches
• Hands behind back stretch
• Hands behind head stretch
• Yawn stretch
• Look over the shoulder stretch
• Calf stretch
• Hip flexor stretch
• Hamstring stretch
• Quadriceps stretch
• Inner hip stretch
• Outer hip stretch

Relaxation

Finish your exercise program by lying down and doing the slow relaxation breathing technique for 1 to 5 minutes. You can also perform Tai Chi or Qi Gong as your cool down.

Nutrition Diary

Design a Safe Kitchen

Your kitchen should be a safe haven, secure from food-borne bacteria contamination. Here is a list of guidelines to set up and maintain your food prep area:

• Use paper towels instead of a dish towel to wipe up after food preparation. This avoids spreading bacteria all over the place.

• Wash all dish towels after two uses. Toss used towels in the wash to keep them out of reach once they've been used twice.

• If your cutting board has been hanging around for 2 or more years, toss it.

• All of this controversy over pots and pans can be confusing. Stainless steel, copper and iron pans generally don't present any health hazards. Any pots or pans with scratches and dents on the surface can be difficult to clean and should go. Toss the old and bring in the new.

Suggested Menu

Have one serving of fruit from the red group such as one half pink grapefruit and one serving of vegetable from the white/green group such as 1 cup fresh mushrooms. Mix the mushrooms with 1 teaspoon olive oil and a shake of garlic powder and top over your sandwich. Try the Yogurt Bowl Recipe for breakfast or a snack.

Breakfast

What I ate _____

_____

What I was doing while I ate

_____

Hunger level: **1**   **2**   **3**   **4**   **5**
　　　　　　　 Full　　　　　　　Starving

Lunch

What I ate _____

_____

What I was doing while I ate

_____

Hunger level: **1**   **2**   **3**   **4**   **5**
　　　　　　　 Full　　　　　　　Starving

Dinner

What I ate _____

_____

What I was doing while I ate

_____

Hunger level: **1**   **2**   **3**   **4**   **5**
　　　　　　　 Full　　　　　　　Starving

Snack (if desired)

What I ate _____

_____

What I was doing while I ate

_____

Hunger level: **1**   **2**   **3**   **4**   **5**
　　　　　　　 Full　　　　　　　Starving

201

Activity Map

Heal Yourself Naturally

Try some of the natural strategies to help you heal and soothe your body and mind.

• Do diaphragmatic breathing.

• Listen to classical music.

• Consider getting a pet.

• Express yourself creatively – sing, dance, write, draw, sculpt.

• Learn to trade massages with your spouse or partner.

• Laugh more.

• Take regular vacations to relieve stress naturally.

• Do some physical activity

• Get enough sleep every night.

• Eat a variety of wholesome and healthy foods.

Warm Up Exercises

Perform all of the following warm up exercises for 1 set of 10 reps for each exercise.

• March in place
• Shake, rattle and roll
• Trunk rotations
• Lower back cat / camel
• Heel sits with arms in front
• Heel sits with arms to side
• Hip windshield wiper

Strength Training Exercises

Perform all of the following muscle building and toning exercises for 1 to 2 sets of 10 to 15 reps at an OMNI RPE of 3 to 4.

• Wall ball squats
• Heel raises
• Partial step-ups
• Elastic pull to chest
• Elastic pull to hips
• Wingspan elastic pulls
• Dumbbell chest press
• Elastic triceps pushdown
• Dumbbell biceps curl
• Supine bridging
• Abdominal bracing
• Floor abdominal curls
• Pelvic floor

Balance Exercises

Perform both balance exercises for 1 set of 30 seconds.

• Very slow motion balancing and walking in place
• Dancer's balance

Stretching Exercises

Perform all of the following stretching exercise for 1 set of 15 to 30 seconds.

• Wrist stretch
• Neck stretches
• Hands behind back stretch
• Hands behind head stretch
• Yawn stretch
• Look over the shoulder stretch
• Calf stretch
• Hip flexor stretch
• Hamstring stretch
• Quadriceps stretch
• Inner hip stretch
• Outer hip stretch

Relaxation

Finish your exercise program by lying down and doing the slow relaxation breathing technique for 1 to 5 minutes. You can also perform Tai Chi or Qi Gong as your cool down.

202

Nutrition Diary

Choosing Meats

To decide what cut of meat to buy, remember lean meat = the healthiest meat. Look for 3 grams of fat per ounce or less. Here is a list of some of the healthier cuts of meat:

- Skinless chicken and turkey, both white and dark meat

- Beef select or choice grades trimmed of fat, filet mignon, round, sirloin, flank steak, tenderloin. Steak: T-bone, porterhouse. Roast: rib, chuck, rump. Ground beef: 90% lean or leaner

- Pork tenderloin, Canadian bacon, ham, pork center loin chop

- Game: Duck or pheasant (no skin), venison, buffalo or ostrich

Suggested Menu

Have one serving fruit from the red/purple group such as 1 cup red grapes and one serving of vegetable from the orange group such as one serving of Spicy Pumpkin Dip. Spread between two slices whole wheat toast. Have ½ cup 1% cottage cheese.

Breakfast

What I ate _____

_____

What I was doing while I ate

_____

Hunger level: **1**   **2**   **3**   **4**   **5**
              Full   Starving

Lunch

What I ate _____

_____

What I was doing while I ate

_____

Hunger level: **1**   **2**   **3**   **4**   **5**
              Full   Starving

Dinner

What I ate _____

_____

What I was doing while I ate

_____

Hunger level: **1**   **2**   **3**   **4**   **5**
              Full   Starving

Snack (if desired)

What I ate _____

_____

What I was doing while I ate

_____

Hunger level: **1**   **2**   **3**   **4**   **5**
              Full   Starving

203

the Anti-Aging Fitness
PRESCRIPTION

Activity Map

Boost Your Immune System

• Keep your stress levels under control.

• Be active and exercise daily.

• Get adequate sleep every night.

• Eat a balanced diet of wholesome foods.

• Meditate to calm your mind.

• Avoid excess alcohol.

• Laugh more. Watch a funny movie or read the comics page. How about catching the zany skits on the TV show "I Love Lucy"?

• See your doctor if you have symptoms of depression or anxiety.

Aerobic Training Exercises

Always start your aerobic activity slowly and gradually progress to your target intensity. Choose one the following aerobic activities and do it for 20 to 25 minutes at an OMNI RPE of 3 to 4.

• Walking (outdoor or indoor)
• Biking (outdoor or indoor)
• Pool walking or exercises or swimming
• Dancing (such as salsa)
• Sports (such as tennis)

Stretching Exercises

Perform all of the following stretching exercises for 1 set of 15 to 30 seconds.

• Wrist stretch
• Neck stretches
• Hands behind back stretch
• Hands behind head stretch
• Yawn stretch
• Look over the shoulder stretch
• Calf stretch
• Hip flexor stretch
• Hamstring stretch
• Quadriceps stretch
• Inner hip stretch
• Outer hip stretch

Relaxation

Finish your exercise program by lying down and doing the slow relaxation breathing technique for 1 to 5 minutes. You can also perform Tai Chi or Qi Gong as your cool down.

Anti-Aging Hint:

Think twice and act once. Your plan determines your success, so make sure it's a good one.

204

Nutrition Diary

Safe Preparation and Cooking Guidelines

Handle raw meat preparation on a separate cutting board away from other ingredients to avoid contamination of bacteria that could be in the raw meat with other foods. Wash hands thoroughly with soap and hot water and dry hands after each time that you handle raw meat and before touching anything. When cooking meat, always test the temperature in the thickest part of the meat.

Here are safe internal temperatures for different types of meat:

Fish: 145°

Ground beef: 160°

Pork: 160°

White meat chicken or turkey: 170°

Dark meat chicken or turkey: 180°

Suggested Menu

Have one serving of fruit from the yellow/green group, such as one cup honeydew cubes and one serving of vegetable from the green group, such as 1 cup fresh broccoli, dipped into two tablespoons light salad dressing. Have one cup low fat fruit flavored yogurt.

Breakfast

What I ate _____

_____

What I was doing while I ate

_____

Hunger level: **1**   **2**   **3**   **4**   **5**
            Full   Starving

Lunch

What I ate _____

_____

What I was doing while I ate

_____

Hunger level: **1**   **2**   **3**   **4**   **5**
            Full   Starving

Dinner

What I ate _____

_____

What I was doing while I ate

_____

Hunger level: **1**   **2**   **3**   **4**   **5**
            Full   Starving

Snack (if desired)

What I ate _____

_____

What I was doing while I ate

_____

Hunger level: **1**   **2**   **3**   **4**   **5**
            Full   Starving

the Anti-Aging Fitness
PRESCRIPTION

Activity Map

Age-Defying Hair Care Tip: Hair Today, Gone Tomorrow

We treat our hair like our archenemy, stripping the color, bleaching, coloring, straightening, curling, perming, braiding, and exposing it to the elements.

• Use a shampoo conditioner formulated for your hair type. Don't know your hair type? Ask your stylist or barber.

• If your hair is very curly or wavy, the oils from your scalp don't travel down the hair shaft, so daily conditioning and infrequent washing may be in order to keep your hair in good shape.

• Wear a hat in the sun. UV rays can damage hair.

Your Bodyweight:_____

From Z and Tracy: We bet that you're feeling good today since your clothes probably feel a little looser. Give us a high five or low five or whatever it is these days. Make sure you change your aerobic activities periodically.

Warm Up Exercises

Perform all of the following warm up exercises for 1 set of 10 reps for each exercise.

- March in place
- Shake, rattle and roll
- Trunk rotations
- Lower back cat / camel
- Heel sits with arms in front
- Heel sits with arms to side
- Hip windshield wiper

Stretching Exercises

Perform all of the following stretching exercises for 1 set of 15 to 30 seconds.

- Wrist stretch
- Neck stretches
- Hands behind back stretch
- Hands behind head stretch
- Yawn stretch
- Look over the shoulder stretch
- Calf stretch
- Hip flexor stretch
- Hamstring stretch
- Quadriceps stretch
- Inner hip stretch
- Outer hip stretch

Relaxation

Finish your exercise program by lying down and doing the slow relaxation breathing technique for 1 to 5 minutes. You can also perform Tai Chi or Qi Gong as your cool down.

Did You Know That...

There are 33 vertebrae, 31 pairs of spinal nerves and 23 intervertebral discs in the spine. Good body mechanics and posture as well as proper nutrition and exercise will help keep these structures healthy and pain free.

Nutrition Diary

the **Anti-Aging Fitness**
PRESCRIPTION

Challenge Yourself: Try Tai Chi

Tai Chi (also known as Tai Chi Ch'uan) is a traditional Chinese martial art where a series of slow controlled movements helps to improve balance, relaxation, mental concentration, flexibility, and strength. Tai Chi is sometimes considered as a mind in action or meditation in motion. Contact a local martial arts studio and take a few classes to see if this is a method you want to further explore.

Suggested Menu

Have one serving fruit from the orange group such as 5 dried apricot halves and one serving of vegetable from the red/purple group such as one half cup canned beets. Make a salad with 1 cup shredded romaine lettuce, topped with ½ cup drained canned beets, 5 apricot halves, and 1 tablespoon balsamic vinaigrette salad dressing. Have one slice soy cheese, such as veggie slices.

Breakfast

What I ate _____

_____

What I was doing while I ate

_____

Hunger level: **1**   **2**   **3**   **4**   **5**
         Full   Starving

Lunch

What I ate _____

_____

What I was doing while I ate

_____

Hunger level: **1**   **2**   **3**   **4**   **5**
         Full   Starving

Dinner

What I ate _____

_____

What I was doing while I ate

_____

Hunger level: **1**   **2**   **3**   **4**   **5**
         Full   Starving

Snack (if desired)

What I ate _____

_____

What I was doing while I ate

_____

Hunger level: **1**   **2**   **3**   **4**   **5**
         Full   Starving

207

the **Anti-Aging Fitness**
PRESCRIPTION

Activity Map

Side Effects Of Obesity

• **Lower Back Pain:** Obesity is associated with lower back pain. So losing weight may help you reduce your back pain.

• **Sleep Disturbance:** Obesity can cause sleep disturbance and is a significant risk factor for sleep apnea.

• **Cancer:** Increased body weight (obesity and being excess body weight) is associated with increased death rates for all cancers combined.

• **Type 2 diabetes (insulin resistance syndrome):** Increasing physical activity can help prevent type 2 diabetes and weight loss can dramatically benefit how a type 2 diabetic manages this disease.

• **Asthma:** Obesity and overweight may be associated with the development of asthma.

From Z and Tracy: Okay now we enter week four. No problem. Think about changing your aerobic activities a little this week. Don't just go for a walk. Why not take a dance class or play a casual game of tennis? This week you'll be continuing to increase the time and intensity of your aerobic exercises and also decreasing the number of repetitions with your strength training exercises but increasing the weight.

Aerobic Training Exercises

Always start your aerobic activity slowly and gradually progress to your target intensity. Choose one the following aerobic activities and do it for 25 to 30 minutes at an OMNI RPE of 4 to 5.

• Walking (outdoor or indoor)
• Biking (outdoor or indoor)
• Pool walking or exercises or swimming
• Dancing (such as salsa)
• Sports (such as tennis)

Stretching Exercises

Perform all of the following stretching exercises for 2 sets of 15 to 30 seconds.

• Wrist stretch
• Neck stretches
• Hands behind back stretch
• Hands behind head stretch
• Yawn stretch
• Look over the shoulder stretch
• Calf stretch
• Hip flexor stretch
• Hamstring stretch
• Quadriceps stretch
• Inner hip stretch
• Outer hip stretch

Relaxation

Finish your exercise program by lying down and doing the slow relaxation breathing technique for 1 to 5 minutes. You can also perform Tai Chi or Qi Gong as your cool down.

Nutrition Diary

Three-A-Day

We've been slowly gearing up to your three-a-day of fruits, vegetables, calcium-rich foods and meals. On Day 22 you move from one vegetable, fruit and calcium-rich food every day to a suggested menu for all meals incorporating the anti-aging recipes. You can follow the suggested menus closely, or you can choose recipes that appeal to you and create your own meal plan (see Mix 'n Match Anti-Aging Meal Plan on page 160).

Breakfast

What I ate _____

_____

What I was doing while I ate

_____

Hunger level: **1**   **2**   **3**   **4**   **5**
              Full   Starving

Lunch

What I ate _____

_____

What I was doing while I ate

_____

Hunger level: **1**   **2**   **3**   **4**   **5**
              Full   Starving

Dinner

What I ate _____

_____

What I was doing while I ate

_____

Hunger level: **1**   **2**   **3**   **4**   **5**
              Full   Starving

Snack (if desired)

What I ate _____

_____

What I was doing while I ate

_____

Hunger level: **1**   **2**   **3**   **4**   **5**
              Full   Starving

Suggested Menu

Breakfast
Have ½ cup cooked oatmeal topped with ½ cup blueberries and 1 tbsp chopped walnuts, 1½ cups fat-free milk, and 1 sliced orange

Lunch
Have 1 6" whole wheat roll topped with one 3-oz chicken breast, ½ cup baby spinach, ¼ cup red onion, 4 slices tomato and ½ sliced yellow bell pepper spread with 1 tbsp light mayonnaise and Dijon mustard. Serve with 1½ cups fat-free milk and ½ cup red grapes

Snack
Have 1 Frozen Milk Pop.

Dinner
Have 1 serving Lemon Lime Salmon with Asparagus. Make whole recipe, save half for dinner Day 24. Serve with 3 oz baked sweet potato topped with 2 tsp light, trans-free margarine and 1 banana topped with 4 tbsp Cool Whip and 1 tbsp slivered almonds.

Daily Calorie total: 1612
Fat, 40 g % of daily cal: 22%
Saturated Fat, 10 g % of daily cal: 6%
Carbohydrate, 217 g % of daily cal: 54%
Protein, 107 g % of daily cal: 27%
Fiber, 30 g
Cholesterol, 157 mg
Calcium, 1209 mg
Sodium, 1196 mg

the**Anti-Aging Fitness**
PRESCRIPTION

Activity Map

Fidgeting To Burn Calories

Studies have shown that non-exercise activity, things people do as a part of daily life, such as fidgeting (tapping your foot or hand, adjusting your sitting position), walking or strolling around, going from sitting to standing, or standing instead of sitting to do tasks, can help you burn calories and assist you in controlling your weight. A study found that obese individuals could burn around 350 calories per day if they were more active during the day and fidgeted more. So don't sit there like a potted plant! Get up and move around and add a little groove to your step and life.

From Z and Tracy: Today we increase your strength training program to 1 to 2 sets of 8 to 12 reps. As you reduce reps, you will be increasing the weights or resistance for your strength exercises. Your balance exercises increase to 1 to 2 sets of 30 seconds.

Warm Up Exercises

Perform all of the following warm up exercises for 1 set of 10 reps for each exercise.

- March in place
- Shake, rattle and roll
- Trunk rotations
- Lower back cat/camel
- Heel sits with arms in front
- Heel sits with arms to side
- Hip windshield wiper

Strength Training Exercises

Perform all of the following muscle building and toning exercises for 1 to 2 sets of 8 to 12 reps at an OMNI RPE of 4 to 5.

- Wall ball squats
- Heel raises
- Partial step-ups
- Elastic pull to chest
- Elastic pull to hips
- Wingspan elastic pulls
- Modified pushups
- Elastic triceps pushdown
- Dumbbell biceps curl
- Supine bridging
- Exercise ball abdominal curls
- Pelvic floor contract, hold, release

Balance Exercises

Perform both balance exercises for 1 to 2 sets of 30 seconds.

- Very slow motion balancing and walking in place
- Dancer's balance

Stretching Exercises

Perform all of the following stretching exercise for 2 sets of 15 to 30 seconds.

- Wrist stretch
- Neck stretches
- Hands behind back stretch
- Hands behind head stretch
- Yawn stretch
- Look over the shoulder stretch
- Calf stretch
- Hip flexor stretch
- Hamstring stretch
- Quadriceps stretch
- Inner hip stretch
- Outer hip stretch

Relaxation

Finish your exercise program by lying down and doing the slow relaxation breathing technique for 1 to 5 minutes. You can also perform Tai Chi or Qi Gong as your cool down.

Nutrition Diary

Freezer Safety Tips

• Always defrost frozen meat in the refrigerator, never in the sink or out on the counter.

• Because long-term freezing can change the taste of spices in a dish, you may choose to add the spices as you reheat the food. Don't forget to note any special directions for preparation on the label.

• Once you've defrosted your meat in the refrigerator, cook the meat within three days. Bacteria will begin to grow more rapidly as it sits in the refrigerator, so the sooner the better. Always freeze leftovers that you won't eat within one day.

Cooked dishes will keep safely in your refrigerator for three days. Don't let any of your precious prepared meals go to waste. If you don't anticipate serving the dish within a day or two, freeze it right away.

Breakfast

What I ate _____

_____

What I was doing while I ate

_____

Hunger level: **1**   **2**   **3**   **4**   **5**
                  Full   Starving

Lunch

What I ate _____

_____

What I was doing while I ate

_____

Hunger level: **1**   **2**   **3**   **4**   **5**
                  Full   Starving

Dinner

What I ate _____

_____

What I was doing while I ate

_____

Hunger level: **1**   **2**   **3**   **4**   **5**
                  Full   Starving

Snack (if desired)

What I ate _____

_____

What I was doing while I ate

_____

Hunger level: **1**   **2**   **3**   **4**   **5**
                  Full   Starving

Suggested Menu

Breakfast
Preheat the oven to 200 degrees, split open one 6" whole wheat pita, fill with 1 slice soy cheese, 1 thinly sliced pear and a sprinkle of cinnamon, heat for 4–5 minutes. Serve with 1 cup fat-free milk.

Lunch
Serve 3 cups baby spinach greens and 1 sliced red bell pepper and top with 2 oz roasted chicken breast, 2 tsp toasted pine nuts and 2 tbsp light ranch dressing. Serve with 1 cup fat-free milk and ½ cup canned chunk pineapple (juice or water pack).

Snack
Have 1 cup low fat plain yogurt topped with ½ sliced mango.

Dinner
Make Turkey Empanadas. Save 1 serving for lunch on Day 24. Serve with a small ear of yellow corn (frozen or fresh). Have 1 fudgesicle.

Daily Calorie total: 1659
Fat, 39 g % of daily cal: 21%
Saturated Fat, 13 g % of daily cal: 7%
Carbohydrate, 230 g % of daily cal: 55%
Protein, 108 g % of daily cal: 26%
Fiber, 27 g
Cholesterol, 185 mg
Calcium, 1400 mg
Sodium, 2251 mg

Activity Map

Instant Exercise with Daily Chores

• Park your car further away from the store to get more daily steps. Every step counts!

• Do slow heel raises, weight shifting from one leg to the other or partial single leg balancing while waiting in line at the grocery store, bank or post office.

• Do mini squats while cooking.

• Weight shift from one leg to the other while doing the dishes.

• Straighten and bend one knee while watching TV and then do the other side.

• Get up and walk in place for one minute after watching TV for 30 minutes.

• Get up and do a "yawn" stretch every 30 minutes while working on your computer.

Aerobic Training Exercises

Always start your aerobic activity slowly and gradually progress to your target intensity. Choose one the following aerobic activities and do it for 25 to 30 minutes at an OMNI RPE of 4 to 5.

• Walking (outdoor or indoor)
• Biking (outdoor or indoor)
• Pool walking or exercises or swimming
• Dancing (such as salsa)
• Sports (such as tennis)

Stretching Exercises

Perform all of the following stretching exercises for 2 sets of 15 to 30 seconds.

• Wrist stretch
• Neck stretches
• Hands behind back stretch
• Hands behind head stretch
• Yawn stretch
• Look over the shoulder stretch
• Calf stretch
• Hip flexor stretch
• Hamstring stretch
• Quadriceps stretch
• Inner hip stretch
• Outer hip stretch

Relaxation

Finish your exercise program by lying down and doing the slow relaxation breathing technique for 1 to 5 minutes. You can also perform Tai Chi or Qi Gong as your cool down.

Nutrition Diary

Make the Best Use of Your Freezer Space

Let's face it. We usually don't know exactly what's in our freezer, nor are we eager to reach in and find out. It's time to throw out any questionable items. If you find something and aren't sure what to do with it, chances are it should be tossed out.

Now that you have some room, here are some guidelines for keeping things safe and orderly.

Start by labeling everything you put in from this point forward with the purchase date. You may use adhesive file labels with a permanent marker or a grease pencil.

After you prepare a dish, the best way to freeze it is to cool it (you can do this in the refrigerator) and wrap it in a dated, freezer-safe, microwave-safe container.

Breakfast

What I ate _____

_____

What I was doing while I ate

_____

Hunger level: **1**   **2**   **3**   **4**   **5**
        Full   Starving

Lunch

What I ate _____

_____

What I was doing while I ate

_____

Hunger level: **1**   **2**   **3**   **4**   **5**
        Full   Starving

Dinner

What I ate _____

_____

What I was doing while I ate

_____

Hunger level: **1**   **2**   **3**   **4**   **5**
        Full   Starving

Snack (if desired)

What I ate _____

_____

What I was doing while I ate

_____

Hunger level: **1**   **2**   **3**   **4**   **5**
        Full   Starving

Suggested Menu

Breakfast

Have 1 serving Fluffy Orange Pancakes. Make whole recipe, save remainder in freezer for breakfast Day 28, 33 and 46. Serve with ½ pink or red grapefruit and 6 oz calcium-fortified orange juice.

Lunch

Have 1 serving Turkey Empanadas leftover from Day 23. Serve with 1½ cups fat-free milk, 1 cup cooked green beans topped with 1 tbsp toasted slivered almonds and ½ mango.

Snack

Have 1 cup sliced strawberries.

Dinner

Have 1 serving Lemon Lime Salmon with Asparagus leftover from Day 22. Serve with 1 serving of Tasty Greens. Make the whole recipe, save half for lunch Day 25. For dessert have 4 Hershey's Kiss candies or 1 fun-size candy bar.

Daily Calorie total: 1602
Fat, 44 g % of daily cal: 25%
Saturated Fat, 11 g % of daily cal: 6%
Carbohydrate, 209 g % of daily cal: 52%
Protein, 104 g % of daily cal: 26%
Fiber, 25 g
Cholesterol, 170 mg
Calcium, 1164 mg
Sodium, 1511 mg

the **Anti-Aging Fitness**
PRESCRIPTION

Activity Map

Step Away Fat

Confucius says that a 1000 mile journey begins with the first step. Well some research has shown that taking 10,000 steps a day (which is about 5 miles) at a fairly fast pace burns about 350-400 calories and is one way of tracking physical activity. 10,000 steps is probably too low for youths and healthy adults while too high for sedentary populations and those with chronic diseases. The key is to keep in mind that the physical activity goal for adults should be to aim for at least 30 minutes of moderate activity on most, if not all, days per week. So you can still take it one step at a time but try to make it brisk, consistent and fun for long term results.

Aerobic Training Exercises

Always start your aerobic activity slowly and gradually progress to your target intensity. Choose one the following aerobic activities and do it for 25 to 30 minutes at an OMNI RPE of 4 to 5.

- Walking (outdoor or indoor)
- Biking (outdoor or indoor)
- Pool walking or exercises or swimming
- Dancing (such as salsa)
- Sports (such as tennis)

Stretching Exercises

Perform all of the following stretching exercises for 2 sets of 15 to 30 seconds.

- Wrist stretch
- Neck stretches
- Hands behind back stretch
- Hands behind head stretch
- Yawn stretch
- Look over the shoulder stretch
- Calf stretch
- Hip flexor stretch
- Hamstring stretch
- Quadriceps stretch
- Inner hip stretch
- Outer hip stretch

Relaxation

Finish your exercise program by lying down and doing the slow relaxation breathing technique for 1 to 5 minutes. You can also perform Tai Chi or Qi Gong as your cool down.

Anti-Aging Hint:

If you want to eat more and weigh less, then focus more on nutritious vegetables.

214

Nutrition Diary

Vegetable Garden in the Freezer

Frozen vegetables are the best kept secret around. They are nutritious (most are frozen within hours of being picked) and last up to six months. Choose Grade A or "fancy" frozen vegetables.

When stir frying frozen vegetables, experiment with different oils and nuts and seeds to pack some flavor into your dishes. For an Asian flair, try sesame oil with sesame seeds, for Cajun, try canola oil with cayenne, and lemon peppers; and for Indian, try canola oil with turmeric or cumin.

Experiment with cooking frozen vegetables in your microwave. Just throw them in a microwave-safe dish and add some nuts (about 1 tablespoon per person is ideal) and heat them up for 90 seconds per cup of vegetables, stir and continue heating in 15 second increments until heated through.

Breakfast

What I ate _____

_____

What I was doing while I ate

_____

Hunger level: **1**   **2**   **3**   **4**   **5**
　　　　　　　Full　　　　　　Starving

Lunch

What I ate _____

_____

What I was doing while I ate

_____

Hunger level: **1**   **2**   **3**   **4**   **5**
　　　　　　　Full　　　　　　Starving

Dinner

What I ate _____

_____

What I was doing while I ate

_____

Hunger level: **1**   **2**   **3**   **4**   **5**
　　　　　　　Full　　　　　　Starving

Snack (if desired)

What I ate _____

_____

What I was doing while I ate

_____

Hunger level: **1**   **2**   **3**   **4**   **5**
　　　　　　　Full　　　　　　Starving

Suggested Menu

Breakfast

Have 1 Fruit and Cheese Foldover. Serve with 1½ cups fat-free milk and 1 cup red grapes.

Lunch

Make a sandwich with 2 slices bread (at least 2 g fiber per slice) top with 2 oz lean roast beef, 3 leaves romaine lettuce, 1 sliced red tomato and spread with 1 tbsp horseradish sauce or light mayonnaise. Serve with a side of Tasty Greens leftover from Day 24.

Snack

Dip 2 graham cracker squares in ⅓ cup Peanutty Ricotta Spread. Make whole recipe and save 2 servings in the refrigerator for Day 26 and Day 28, and freeze remainder for Day 50, 51 and 52. Serve with 1 fresh tangerine.

Dinner

Have 1 serving Stoplight Pasta (make whole recipe, save half for Day 26). Serve with 1 cup cooked carrots topped with 2 tsp light trans-free margarine. For dessert, have 1 low fat ice cream sandwich.

Daily Calorie total: 1590
Fat, 41 g % of daily cal: 23%
Saturated Fat, 12 g % of daily cal: 7%
Carbohydrate, 209 g % of daily cal: 53%
Protein, 86 g % of daily cal: 22%
Fiber, 34 g
Cholesterol, 89 mg
Calcium, 1573 mg
Sodium, 2407

the**Anti-Aging Fitness**
PRESCRIPTION

Activity Map

Walk In A Variety of Locations

• Your neighborhood.
• Your local high school or college track.
• Your local park.
• In a shopping mall.
• At the beach if you live near the ocean or a lake.
• At a mountain trail.
• On a treadmill in your home.

Warm Up Exercises

Perform all of the following warm up exercises for 1 set of 10 reps for each exercise.

• March in place
• Shake, rattle and roll
• Trunk rotations
• Lower back cat / camel
• Heel sits with arms in front
• Heel sits with arms to side
• Hip windshield wiper

Strength Training Exercises

Perform all of the following muscle building and toning exercises for 1 to 2 sets of 8 to 12 reps at an OMNI RPE of 4 to 5.

• Wall ball squats
• Heel raises
• Partial step-ups
• Elastic pull to chest
• Elastic pull to hips
• Wingspan elastic pulls
• Modified pushups
• Elastic triceps pushdown
• Dumbbell biceps curl
• Supine bridging
• Exercise ball abdominal curls
• Pelvic floor contract, hold, release

Balance Exercises

Perform both balance exercises for 1 to 2 sets of 30 seconds.

• Very slow motion balancing and walking in place
• Dancer's balance

Stretching Exercises

Perform all of the following stretching exercise for 2 sets of 15 to 30 seconds.

• Wrist stretch
• Neck stretches
• Hands behind back stretch
• Hands behind head stretch
• Yawn stretch
• Look over the shoulder stretch
• Calf stretch
• Hip flexor stretch
• Hamstring stretch
• Quadriceps stretch
• Inner hip stretch
• Outer hip stretch

Relaxation

Finish your exercise program by lying down and doing the slow relaxation breathing technique for 1 to 5 minutes. You can also perform Tai Chi or Qi Gong as your cool down.

One Minute Motivator:

Tis an old saying, That an Ounce of Prevention is Worth a Pound of Cure.
—Benjamin Franklin

216

Nutrition Diary

Try Gardening

Gardening is a simple and practical way of getting some physical activity and at the same time getting some fresh air and sunshine. Gardening can involve raking, digging, carrying, lifting, bending, squatting, kneeling and hand dexterity. It is a peaceful activity. Some people think it's better than meditating in a room. And of course, when you plant a vegetable garden, you get to eat what your efforts produce. You can also save money at the grocery store.

Breakfast

What I ate _____

_____

What I was doing while I ate

_____

Hunger level: **1   2   3   4   5**
           Full   Starving

Lunch

What I ate _____

_____

What I was doing while I ate

_____

Hunger level: **1   2   3   4   5**
           Full   Starving

Dinner

What I ate _____

_____

What I was doing while I ate

_____

Hunger level: **1   2   3   4   5**
           Full   Starving

Snack (if desired)

What I ate _____

_____

What I was doing while I ate

_____

Hunger level: **1   2   3   4   5**
           Full   Starving

Suggested Menu

Breakfast

Spread one 6" whole wheat pita with 8 tbsp Sweet Cream Spread and fill with 6 dried apricots and 1 tbsp raisins. Serve with 1½ cups fat-free milk.

Lunch

Have 1 serving of Stoplight Pasta leftover from dinner Day 25. Serve with 1 small yellow squash sliced and dip in 2 tbsp light salad dressing.

Snack

Toast 1 whole wheat English muffin and top with 1 serving of Peanutty Ricotta spread. Serve with 1 cup fresh cherries or strawberries.

Dinner

Have 1 serving (make ½ of recipe) of Asian Mixed Green Salad with mandarin oranges instead of persimmons. For dessert, have ½ cup of ice cream topped with 2 tbsp whipped topping and 1 tbsp slivered almonds.

Daily Calorie total: 1545
Fat, 39 g % of daily cal: 23%
Saturated Fat, 15 g % of daily cal: 9%
Carbohydrate, 232 g % of daily cal: 60%
Protein, 94 g % of daily cal: 24%
Fiber, 27 g
Cholesterol, 158 mg
Calcium, 1428 mg
Sodium, 2784 mg

the**Anti-Aging Fitness**
PRESCRIPTION

Activity Map

Ways To Vary Your Workouts

• Change Music: Vary what you hear to change the tempo.

• Change Location: Vary your surroundings by going from your living room to the patio or backyard or to a nearby park.

• Change Exercises: Vary the order of exercises.

• Change Time: Vary the time of day you exercise.

• Change Leaders: If you train with a partner then alternate being the one who leads.

• Change Parameters: Change the number of sets, reps, rest periods, intensity.

Aerobic Training Exercises

Always start your aerobic activity slowly and gradually progress to your target intensity. Choose one the following aerobic activities and do it for 25 to 30 minutes at an OMNI RPE of 4 to 5.

• Walking (outdoor or indoor)
• Biking (outdoor or indoor)
• Pool walking or exercises or swimming
• Dancing (such as salsa)
• Sports (such as tennis)

Stretching Exercises

Perform all of the following stretching exercises for 2 sets of 15 to 30 seconds.

• Wrist stretch
• Neck stretches
• Hands behind back stretch
• Hands behind head stretch
• Yawn stretch
• Look over the shoulder stretch
• Calf stretch
• Hip flexor stretch
• Hamstring stretch
• Quadriceps stretch
• Inner hip stretch
• Outer hip stretch

Relaxation

Finish your exercise program by lying down and doing the slow relaxation breathing technique for 1 to 5 minutes. You can also perform Tai Chi or Qi Gong as your cool down.

218

Nutrition Diary

Your Friend Fiber

Fiber is an important component of your diet, but especially those with high blood cholesterol or diabetes. Both soluble and insoluble fibers slow starch breakdown and delay glucose absorption into the bloodstream.

Soluble: Found in oat, fruit, barley, vegetables and legumes.

• Delays stomach emptying.

• Lowers blood cholesterol level.

Insoluble: Found in vegetables, whole-grain products and cereals.

• Speeds contents through the small intestine.

Suggested Menu

Breakfast
Have 1 serving of Yogurt Bowl.
Lunch
Make a grilled cheese sandwich with 1 slice soy cheese and spread outsides of each slice whole wheat bread with 1 tbsp light trans-free margarine (total). Preheat a small skillet coated with cooking spray over medium heat and grill. Serve with 1 cup sweet green peas and a peach.
Snack
Serve 1 cup watermelon cubes and 8 whole almonds.
Dinner
Have 1 serving Chili (Make whole recipe, save 2 servings for Days 29 and 30 and freeze one serving for Day 55). Serve with a side of 1 cup cooked broccoli florets topped with 1 tbsp of light, trans-free margarine. For dessert, have 1 fudgesicle.

Daily Calorie total: 1573
Fat, 35 g % of daily cal: 20%
Saturated Fat, 9 g % of daily cal: 5%
Carbohydrate, 244 g % of daily cal: 63%
Protein, 91 g % of daily cal: 23%
Fiber, 51 g
Cholesterol, 65 mg
Calcium, 1201 mg
Sodium, 1800 mg

Breakfast

What I ate _____

_____

What I was doing while I ate

_____

Hunger level: **1   2   3   4   5**
　　　　　Full　　　　Starving

Lunch

What I ate _____

_____

What I was doing while I ate

_____

Hunger level: **1   2   3   4   5**
　　　　　Full　　　　Starving

Dinner

What I ate _____

_____

What I was doing while I ate

_____

Hunger level: **1   2   3   4   5**
　　　　　Full　　　　Starving

Snack (if desired)

What I ate _____

_____

What I was doing while I ate

_____

Hunger level: **1   2   3   4   5**
　　　　　Full　　　　Starving

219

Activity Map

The Art of the Perfect Shave

• Make sure your skin is wet for 1 to 2 minutes before shaving. Wait until after your shower or bath.

• Experiment to find a razor (or an electric shaver) that works well on your skin.

• Experiment to find a non-irritating shave gel.

• To avoid irritation, don't shave against the growth of the hair (go with the grain). Avoid repeat strokes in the same area to prevent irritation.

• After shaving, gently splash your skin with cool water and then pat dry with a soft cotton towel.

Your Bodyweight:_____

From Z and Tracy: You just completed 4 weeks. Go do something fun today. You truly deserve it. Drop hints with your partner to take you out for a fun night. None of this sitting in front of a TV. So hide the remote and go decide what you want to wear. See you tomorrow.

Warm Up Exercises

Perform all of the following warm up exercises for 1 set of 10 reps for each exercise.

• March in place
• Shake, rattle and roll
• Trunk rotations
• Lower back cat / camel

• Heel sits with arms in front
• Heel sits with arms to side
• Hip windshield wiper

Stretching Exercises

Perform all of the following stretching exercise for 2 sets of 15 to 30 seconds.

• Wrist stretch
• Neck stretches
• Hands behind back stretch
• Hands behind head stretch
• Yawn stretch
• Look over the shoulder stretch

• Calf stretch
• Hip flexor stretch
• Hamstring stretch
• Quadriceps stretch
• Inner hip stretch
• Outer hip stretch

Relaxation

Finish your exercise program by lying down and doing the slow relaxation breathing technique for 1 to 5 minutes. You can also perform Tai Chi or Qi Gong as your cool down.

Did You Know That...

The brain accounts for only 2% of an adult's body weight. However, at any given time the brain contains 15% of the body's blood, and it uses 20 to 30% of the fuel that supports the basal metabolism. During increased brain activity, neuronal metabolism can increase as much as an extra 100 to 150%. So feed your mind good nutrition to keep you functioning at peak levels. It might even help you get that raise you were looking for at work!

Nutrition Diary

Revisiting Your Goals

Back on Day 7, you mapped out some goals. How are you doing? Have you introduced new foods or new activity to your day? Create some goals that include some of your new healthy lifestyle changes.

I plan to follow these steps to better health ...

1. _____
2. _____
3. _____

Breakfast

What I ate _____

_____

What I was doing while I ate

_____

Hunger level: **1   2   3   4   5**
  Full   Starving

Lunch

What I ate _____

_____

What I was doing while I ate

_____

Hunger level: **1   2   3   4   5**
              Full   Starving

Dinner

What I ate _____

_____

What I was doing while I ate

_____

Hunger level: **1   2   3   4   5**
  Full   Starving

Snack (if desired)

What I ate _____

_____

What I was doing while I ate

_____

Hunger level: **1   2   3   4   5**
              Full   Starving

Reward Time

Take advantage of a reward for your efforts!

Suggested Menu

Breakfast
Spread 1 serving of Peanuty Ricotta Spread in an 8" whole wheat soft tortilla, roll up to eat. Serve with 1 cup fat-free milk and 1 cup cantaloupe cubes.

Lunch
Make ½ of the Creamy Tomato Soup. Serve with 1 red apple and 1 fresh, sliced yellow pepper, dip into 4 tbsp hummus.

Snack
Have 1 serving Fluffy Orange Pancakes with 1 cup fat-free milk.

Dinner
Have 1 serving Spring Green Walnut Salad. (Make the whole recipe, save 1 serving for Day 29.) For dessert, have ½ cup of ice cream topped with 2 tbsp whipped topping and 1 tbsp slivered almonds.

Daily Calorie total: 1592
Fat, 59 g % of daily cal: 16%
Saturated Fat, 18 g % of daily cal: 10%
Carbohydrate, 207 g % of daily cal: 52%
Protein, 71 g % of daily cal: 18%
Fiber, 33 g
Cholesterol, 194 mg
Calcium, 1406 mg
Sodium, 1726 mg

221

the Anti-Aging Fitness
PRESCRIPTION

Activity Map

Understanding Your Fitness Personality

To get the most out of a fitness program take some time and figure out where you fit best and what you want out of your program.

• Are you looking to be alone with your thoughts? Then try walking or running alone.

• Are you looking for competition? Then try tennis, golf.

• Are you looking for social interaction? Then try dance, or walking with a friend.

• Do you want to relax? Then try Yoga, Tai Chi, Qi Gong, Feldenkrais, or the Alexander Technique.

• Do you want to get physical? Then try weights, martial arts.

• Are you looking for adventure? Then try mountain biking.

From Z and Tracy: This week we're upping your aerobic time to 30 to 40 minutes and you'll be doing your cardio workout 5 times this week. Before you think about it too much, please go get your workout gear and let's get moving.

Aerobic Training Exercises

Always start your aerobic activity slowly and gradually progress to your target intensity. Choose one the following aerobic activities and do it for 30 to 40 minutes at an OMNI RPE of 5 to 6.

• Walking (outdoor or indoor)
• Biking (outdoor or indoor)
• Pool walking or exercises or swimming

• Dancing (such as salsa)
• Sports (such as tennis)

Stretching Exercises

Perform all of the following stretching exercises for 2 sets of 15 to 30 seconds.

• Wrist stretch
• Neck stretches
• Hands behind back stretch
• Hands behind head stretch
• Yawn stretch
• Look over the shoulder stretch

• Calf stretch
• Hip flexor stretch
• Hamstring stretch
• Quadriceps stretch
• Inner hip stretch
• Outer hip stretch

Relaxation

Finish your exercise program by lying down and doing the slow relaxation breathing technique for 1 to 5 minutes. You can also perform Tai Chi or Qi Gong as your cool down.

222

Nutrition Diary

Get a Handle on Comfort Eating

Traffic is bumper to bumper and you arrive at work 20 minutes late, which means you'll have to stay late to make up the time. You start snacking on a bag of Fig Newtons. By the end of the day, you realize you've eaten three quarters of the bag! Now you feel bloated and guilty for overeating, and the last thing you want to do is go work out.

You can regain control. The key is to replace eating with another activity that gives you comfort.

- Fill your MP3 player with your favorite music, and keep it nearby.
- Call a family member or friend and catch up on what's new.
- Sip a cold, flavored seltzer water with a straw.
- Read 10 pages of a book you've been dying to read.

Breakfast

What I ate _____

_____

What I was doing while I ate

_____

Hunger level: **1**   **2**   **3**   **4**   **5**
          Full   Starving

Lunch

What I ate _____

_____

What I was doing while I ate

_____

Hunger level: **1**   **2**   **3**   **4**   **5**
          Full   Starving

Dinner

What I ate _____

_____

What I was doing while I ate

_____

Hunger level: **1**   **2**   **3**   **4**   **5**
          Full   Starving

Snack (if desired)

What I ate _____

_____

What I was doing while I ate

_____

Hunger level: **1**   **2**   **3**   **4**   **5**
          Full   Starving

Suggested Menu

Breakfast

Have 1 serving Spicy Pumpkin Dip. (Make ½ of recipe, freeze 1 serving for Day 53 and refrigerate 1 serving for Day 30) with 1 slice toasted cinnamon raisin bread. Serve with 1 cup cut honeydew and 1 cup fat-free milk.

Lunch

Have 1 serving Spring Green Walnut Salad. Serve with 1 cup low fat vanilla yogurt.

Snack

Make 1 serving (¼ of recipe) of Layered Dip and Tortilla Chips. Serve with 1 cup fat-free milk.

Dinner

Have one serving of Chili leftover from Day 27. Serve with 1½ cups cooked broccoli, cauliflower and carrot mixture topped with 1 tbsp light, trans-free margarine. For dessert, have 1 low-fat ice cream sandwich.

Daily Calorie total: 1610
Fat, 38 g %of daily cal: 21%
Saturated Fat, 7 g %of daily cal: 4%
Carbohydrate, 252 g %of daily cal: 62%
Protein, 77 g %of daily cal: 19%
Fiber, 51 g
Cholesterol, 57 mg
Calcium, 1420 mg
Sodium, 1945 mg

Activity Map

Osteoporosis and Exercise Tips

If you have osteoporosis, consult with your doctor and physical therapist so they can discuss the following with you:

- Good posture
- Body mechanics
- Weight training
- Dance class
- Tai Chi
- Aerobic exercises such as walking (you might want to use a weighted vest while walking)
- Sports such as tennis
- Doing 1 to 2 deep breaths once a day while seated in a chair. Avoid too many breaths to prevent dizziness.

From Z and Tracy: This week we increase your strength program to 2 sets of 8 to 12 reps, your stretching program to 2 sets of 15 to 30 seconds and finally, your balance exercises to 1 to 2 sets of 30 to 60 seconds.

Warm Up Exercises

Perform all of the following warm up exercises for 1 set of 10 reps for each exercise.

- March in place
- Shake, rattle and roll
- Trunk rotations
- Lower back cat / camel
- Heel sits with arms in front
- Heel sits with arms to side
- Hip windshield wiper

Strength Training Exercises

Perform all of the following muscle building and toning exercises for 2 sets of 8 to 12 reps at an OMNI RPE of 5 to 6.

- Wall ball squats
- Heel raises
- Partial step-ups
- Elastic pull to chest
- Elastic outward rotation
- Dumbbell overhead press
- Modified pushups
- Elastic triceps pushdown
- Dumbbell biceps curl
- Supine bridging
- Exercise ball abdominal curls
- Pelvic floor contract, hold, release

Balance Exercises

Perform both balance exercises for 1 to 2 sets of 30 to 60 seconds.

- Very slow motion balancing and walking in place
- Dancer's balance

Stretching Exercises

Perform all of the following stretching exercises for 2 sets of 15 to 30 seconds.

- Wrist stretch
- Neck stretches
- Hands behind back stretch
- Hands behind head stretch
- Yawn stretch
- Look over the shoulder stretch
- Calf stretch
- Hip flexor stretch
- Hamstring stretch
- Quadriceps stretch
- Inner hip stretch
- Outer hip stretch

Relaxation

Finish your exercise program by lying down and doing the slow relaxation breathing technique for 1 to 5 minutes. You can also perform Tai Chi or Qi Gong as your cool down.

224

Nutrition Diary

Your Support Network

Use your support network. To stay on track, include your friends and family in your new eating and exercise plan and steer clear of negative influences from other people.

Don't allow anyone to sabotage your efforts to improve your health. Sometimes a spouse or friend is threatened by your new physique or the energy that comes from a new eating and exercise program. Involve your loved ones in your progress as much as you can.

You are responsible for your own success. No one can derail you unless you allow it.

Breakfast

What I ate _____

_____

What I was doing while I ate

_____

Hunger level: **1**   **2**   **3**   **4**   **5**
                Full   Starving

Lunch

What I ate _____

_____

What I was doing while I ate

_____

Hunger level: **1**   **2**   **3**   **4**   **5**
                Full   Starving

Dinner

What I ate _____

_____

What I was doing while I ate

_____

Hunger level: **1**   **2**   **3**   **4**   **5**
                Full   Starving

Snack (if desired)

What I ate _____

_____

What I was doing while I ate

_____

Hunger level: **1**   **2**   **3**   **4**   **5**
                Full   Starving

Suggested Menu

Breakfast
Toast 1 whole wheat English muffin topped with 1½ slices soy cheese. Serve with 1 plum, 1 kiwi, 1 cup fat-free milk and 1 cup fruit-flavored yogurt.

Lunch
Have 1 serving of Chili leftover from Day 27. Serve with 1 cup watermelon cubes.

Snack
Have 1 serving of Spicy Pumpkin Dip leftover from Day 29. Serve with 4 squares graham crackers.

Dinner
Have 1 serving Beef, Broccoli and Tomatoes. (Make entire recipe, save 1 serving for Day 32). Serve with 1 Frozen Milk Pop.

Daily Calorie total: 1591
Fat, 30 g % of daily cal: 17%
Saturated Fat, 10 g % of daily cal: 6%
Carbohydrate, 239 g % of daily cal: 60%
Protein, 103 g % of daily cal: 26%
Fiber, 27 g
Cholesterol, 119 mg
Calcium, 1468 mg
Sodium, 1631 mg

225

the**Anti-Aging Fitness**
PRESCRIPTION

Activity Map

Arthritis and Exercise Tips

If you have arthritis, consult with your doctor and physical therapist about the following:

• Exercise to help improve your strength, flexibility, range of motion, and endurance.

• Exercise on surfaces that decrease joint impact.

• Wearing good walking shoes that are supportive.

• Alternate sports and activities to reduce placing the same physical stress on the joints.

• Maintaining ideal body weight.

Anti-Aging Hint:

Variety is the spice of life. So vary your activities for more fun. Take classes to learn new activities or sports to challenge yourself.

Aerobic Training Exercises

Always start your aerobic activity slowly and gradually progress to your target intensity. Choose one the following aerobic activities and do it for 30 to 40 minutes at an OMNI RPE of 5 to 6.

• Walking (outdoor or indoor)
• Biking (outdoor or indoor)
• Pool walking or exercises or swimming
• Dancing (such as salsa)
• Sports (such as tennis)

Stretching Exercises

Perform all of the following stretching exercises for 2 sets of 15 to 30 seconds.

• Wrist stretch
• Neck stretches
• Hands behind back stretch
• Hands behind head stretch
• Yawn stretch
• Look over the shoulder stretch
• Calf stretch
• Hip flexor stretch
• Hamstring stretch
• Quadriceps stretch
• Inner hip stretch
• Outer hip stretch

Relaxation

Finish your exercise program by lying down and doing the slow relaxation breathing technique for 1 to 5 minutes. You can also perform Tai Chi or Qi Gong as your cool down.

226

Nutrition Diary

Urban Legend from the World of Nutrition

"I'm addicted to sweets! There's no way for me to ever stop eating candy."

Sweets typically have very little protein and fat, with the exception of chocolate candy, so your blood glucose raises substantially and quickly with sweets. Sometimes we become so accustomed to the rise in blood glucose and the endorphin release that can accompany this rise, that we think we're addicted. There is caffeine in chocolate, but not enough to trigger a need for caffeine. Instead, have one treat every day, limit the portion and have your treat with a meal, as we suggest, or pair it with a few tablespoons of nuts to provide a little protein to keep your blood sugar from skyrocketing, and then dropping, leaving you hungry for more.

Breakfast

What I ate _____

_____

What I was doing while I ate

_____

Hunger level: **1**   **2**   **3**   **4**   **5**
                Full   Starving

Lunch

What I ate _____

_____

What I was doing while I ate

_____

Hunger level: **1**   **2**   **3**   **4**   **5**
                Full   Starving

Dinner

What I ate _____

_____

What I was doing while I ate

_____

Hunger level: **1**   **2**   **3**   **4**   **5**
                Full   Starving

Snack (if desired)

What I ate _____

_____

What I was doing while I ate

_____

Hunger level: **1**   **2**   **3**   **4**   **5**
                Full   Starving

Suggested Menu

Breakfast
Toast 2 whole grain waffles, top with ½ cup 1% cottage cheese and 1 cup frozen, unsweetened strawberries. Serve with 1½ cups fat-free milk.

Lunch
Have 1 serving Grapefruit Salad with Salmon. (Make ½ of recipe.)

Snack
Have 1 serving of Creamy Tomato Soup leftover from Day 28.

Dinner
Have 1 serving Lime Peanut Salad. (Make entire recipe, save ½ for Day 32.) Serve with 1 banana. For dessert, have 1 Pria bar.

Daily Calorie total: 1550
Fat, 52 g % of daily cal: 30%
Saturated Fat, 13 g % of daily cal: 8%
Carbohydrate, 223 g % of daily cal: 58%
Protein, 66 g % of daily cal: 17%
Fiber, 27 g
Cholesterol, 154 mg
Calcium, 1377 mg
Sodium, 2816 mg

227

the **Anti-Aging Fitness**
PRESCRIPTION

Activity Map

Premenstrual Syndrome (PMS): Easing The Discomfort

Women with PMS can have a variety of symptoms such as tension, irritability, depression, anxiety, mood swings, cravings for sugar, sleep disturbance, abdominal bloating and swelling.

An article in the *Canadian Family Physician* and the *American Journal of Obstetrics and Gynecology* outline some simple self-help methods that may ease the symptoms of PMS: getting adequate enough calcium in the diet, eating a diet rich in complex carbohydrates, doing aerobic exercise, getting enough sleep, reducing stress with relaxation techniques and reducing caffeine. If those don't do the trick, then see your physician.

Aerobic Training Exercises

Always start your aerobic activity slowly and gradually progress to your target intensity. Choose one the following aerobic activities and do it for 30 to 40 minutes at an OMNI RPE of 5 to 6.

- Walking (outdoor or indoor)
- Biking (outdoor or indoor)
- Pool walking or exercises or swimming
- Dancing (such as salsa)
- Sports (such as tennis)

Stretching Exercises

Perform all of the following stretching exercises for 2 sets of 15 to 30 seconds.

- Wrist stretch
- Neck stretches
- Hands behind back stretch
- Hands behind head stretch
- Yawn stretch
- Look over the shoulder stretch
- Calf stretch
- Hip flexor stretch
- Hamstring stretch
- Quadriceps stretch
- Inner hip stretch
- Outer hip stretch

Relaxation

Finish your exercise program by lying down and doing the slow relaxation breathing technique for 1 to 5 minutes. You can also perform Tai Chi or Qi Gong as your cool down.

Nutrition Diary

Practical Weight Loss Tips

• Chart your progress in a journal, diary or log as you are doing here in our 8-week plan.

• Work out with a training partner for motivation.

• Plan your day around your health first. Know what you're going to eat for breakfast, lunch, and dinner. Also plan when you will exercise and what time you will go to sleep.

• Set realistic goals that you want to accomplish.

• Create a rewards program for yourself for being able to lose weight and maintain the weight loss.

• Perform stretching, calisthenics, and light weight training while you watch your favorite television shows

• Take active vacations that involve walking, hiking, canoeing, and bicycling.

Breakfast

What I ate _____

_____

What I was doing while I ate

_____

Hunger level: **1   2   3   4   5**
         Full   Starving

Lunch

What I ate _____

_____

What I was doing while I ate

_____

Hunger level: **1   2   3   4   5**
         Full   Starving

Dinner

What I ate _____

_____

What I was doing while I ate

_____

Hunger level: **1   2   3   4   5**
         Full   Starving

Snack (if desired)

What I ate _____

_____

What I was doing while I ate

_____

Hunger level: **1   2   3   4   5**
         Full   Starving

Suggested Menu

Breakfast
Have 1 Crunchy Banana Pop. (Make entire recipe, save 1 serving for a snack on Day 33. Serve with 1½ cups flavored low fat soy milk.

Lunch
Have 1 serving Beef, Broccoli and Tomatoes leftover from Day 30. Serve with 1 cup cantaloupe cubes.

Snack
Make 1 Very Berry Smoothie, use blackberries.

Dinner
Have 1 serving of Lime Peanut Salad leftover from Day 31. For dessert, have 3 store-bought meringue cookies.

Daily Calorie total: 1604
Fat, 59 g % of daily cal: 33%
Saturated Fat, 18 g % of daily cal: 10%
Carbohydrate, 198 g % of daily cal: 49%
Protein, 89 g % of daily cal: 22%
Fiber, 51 g
Cholesterol, 94 mg
Calcium, 1478 mg
Sodium, 1424 mg

the **Anti-Aging Fitness**
PRESCRIPTION

Activity Map

Menopause: Safe Passage With A Healthy Lifestyle?

Healthy lifestyle changes can significantly influence a woman's overall health and reduce risk of all major diseases and also help the way they feel in general. Healthy changes in diet (such as eating low saturated fat, getting adequate calcium and vitamin D, vitamin K and increased fruits and vegetables), reducing caffeine and alcohol intake, not smoking, exercising, getting adequate sleep, controlling stress and educational supports groups can all make menopause a time to enjoy your accomplishments up to that point in life.

Warm Up Exercises

Perform all of the following warm up exercises for 1 set of 10 reps for each exercise.

- March in place
- Shake, rattle and roll
- Trunk rotations
- Lower back cat/camel
- Heel sits with arms in front
- Heel sits with arms to side
- Hip windshield wiper

Strength Training Exercises

Perform all of the following muscle building and toning exercises for 2 sets of 8 to 12 reps at an OMNI RPE of 5 to 6.

- Wall ball squats
- Heel raises
- Partial step-ups
- Elastic pull to chest
- Elastic outward rotation
- Dumbbell overhead press
- Modified pushups
- Elastic triceps pushdown
- Dumbbell biceps curl
- Supine bridging
- Exercise ball abdominal curls
- Pelvic floor contract, hold, release

Balance Exercises

Perform both balance exercises for 1 to 2 sets of 30 to 60 seconds.

- Very slow motion balancing and walking in place
- Dancer's balance

Stretching Exercises

Perform all of the following stretching exercise for 2 sets of 15 to 30 seconds.

- Wrist stretch
- Neck stretches
- Hands behind back stretch
- Hands behind head stretch
- Yawn stretch
- Look over the shoulder stretch
- Calf stretch
- Hip flexor stretch
- Hamstring stretch
- Quadriceps stretch
- Inner hip stretch
- Outer hip stretch

Relaxation

Finish your exercise program by lying down and doing the slow relaxation breathing technique for 1 to 5 minutes. You can also perform Tai Chi or Qi Gong as your cool down.

230

Nutrition Diary

Tips on Trouncing Those Pounds for Good

- Use smaller plates. You may find it easier to be satisfied with smaller portions.
- Don't supersize. More food is not what you need.
- Don't skip meals. Meal skipping can make you so hungry that you lose your judgment to choose healthy foods when it's time to eat.
- Know your triggers for overeating and plan healthy, low-calorie snacks to have on hand instead of sugary, fatty comfort foods.
- Plan your meals ahead of time to avoid last minute poor choices.
- Don't deny every craving. Avoiding the foods you crave can cause binge eating. Have a little of what you really want. If it sets off a flurry of eating too much of your special food, then choose a different treat.

Breakfast

What I ate _____

_____

What I was doing while I ate

_____

Hunger level: **1**   **2**   **3**   **4**   **5**
　　　　　Full　　　　　　Starving

Lunch

What I ate _____

_____

What I was doing while I ate

_____

Hunger level: **1**   **2**   **3**   **4**   **5**
　　　　　Full　　　　　　Starving

Dinner

What I ate _____

_____

What I was doing while I ate

_____

Hunger level: **1**   **2**   **3**   **4**   **5**
　　　　　Full　　　　　　Starving

Snack (if desired)

What I ate _____

_____

What I was doing while I ate

_____

Hunger level: **1**   **2**   **3**   **4**   **5**
　　　　　Full　　　　　　Starving

Suggested Menu

Breakfast
Have 1 cup low-fat plain yogurt mixed with 1 cup strawberries and 1 tbsp chopped walnuts.

Lunch
Have 1 serving of Black Bean Tomato Bruschetta. (Make ½ of recipe.) Serve with 10 baby carrots.

Snack
Have 1 Crunchy Banana Pop leftover from Day 32. Serve with 1 cup flavored low fat soy milk.

Dinner
Have 1 serving Chicken Mango Salad. (Make the whole recipe, save ½ for Day 34.) For dessert, have 4 Hershey's kiss candies.

Daily Calorie total: 1575
Fat, 41 g % of daily cal: 23%
Saturated Fat, 7 g % of daily cal: 4%
Carbohydrate, 243 g % of daily cal: 62%
Protein, 77 g % of daily cal: 20%
Fiber, 37 g
Cholesterol, 79 mg
Calcium, 1304 mg
Sodium, 1440 mg

231

the**Anti-Aging Fitness**
PRESCRIPTION

Activity Map

Overcoming Plateaus

There you are making nice steady progress in your program and then all of a sudden you're not noticing any more improvement. The following are some tips to get you back on the right track:

• Change nothing and be patient as your body slowly adapts to the changes.

• Take a break for 1 to 2 weeks from your routine and just focus on your non-activity related hobbies.

• Take a vacation. Your mind and body may need a break.

• Make sure you are not overtraining. Back off for recovery.

• Make sure you're getting enough sleep every night.

• Try varying your exercise program.

Aerobic Training Exercises

Always start your aerobic activity slowly and gradually progress to your target intensity. Choose one the following aerobic activities and do it for 30 to 40 minutes at an OMNI RPE of 5 to 6.

• Walking (outdoor or indoor)
• Biking (outdoor or indoor)
• Pool walking or exercises or swimming
• Dancing (such as salsa)
• Sports (such as tennis)

Stretching Exercises

Perform all of the following stretching exercises for 2 sets of 15 to 30 seconds.

• Wrist stretch
• Neck stretches
• Hands behind back stretch
• Hands behind head stretch
• Yawn stretch
• Look over the shoulder stretch
• Calf stretch
• Hip flexor stretch
• Hamstring stretch
• Quadriceps stretch
• Inner hip stretch
• Outer hip stretch

Relaxation

Finish your exercise program by lying down and doing the slow relaxation breathing technique for 1 to 5 minutes. You can also perform Tai Chi or Qi Gong as your cool down.

232

Nutrition Diary

Alcohol and Weight Loss

Alcohol goes down easy and it can be hard to gauge how much you actually drink while you're at a party or enjoying a bottle of wine with a meal. Excess alcohol can play havoc with your ability to lose weight. Alcohol loosens your inhibitions and you may find that you're eating more calories when you've had alcohol. Also, alcohol suppresses the oxidation or burning of fat and, to a lesser degree, that of carbohydrates and protein. In other words, alcohol has a fat-sparing effect and can cause fat gain when consumed in excess of normal energy needs. So limit the amount you drink by filling your glass once and then switch to sparkling water.

Breakfast

What I ate _____

_____

What I was doing while I ate

_____

Hunger level: **1**   **2**   **3**   **4**   **5**
              Full   Starving

Lunch

What I ate _____

_____

What I was doing while I ate

_____

Hunger level: **1**   **2**   **3**   **4**   **5**
              Full   Starving

Dinner

What I ate _____

_____

What I was doing while I ate

_____

Hunger level: **1**   **2**   **3**   **4**   **5**
              Full   Starving

Snack (if desired)

What I ate _____

_____

What I was doing while I ate

_____

Hunger level: **1**   **2**   **3**   **4**   **5**
              Full   Starving

Suggested Menu

Breakfast
Have 1 cup low-fat vanilla yogurt topped with 1 sliced nectarine and 2 tbsp low fat granola. Serve with 1 stick of string cheese.

Lunch
Have 1 serving Chicken Mango Salad leftover from Day 33.

Snack
Have 1 serving Baked Acorn Squash. (Make whole recipe; save ½ for Day 35.) Serve with 1½ cups fat-free milk.

Dinner
Have 1 serving of Pizza with Roasted Vegetables. (Make whole recipe, save 2 servings in the refrigerator for Days 35 and 36 and freeze 1 for Day 56). Serve with 1 cup of honeydew. For dessert, have 1 fudgesicle.

Daily Calorie total: 1588
Fat, 36 g % of daily cal: 20%
Saturated Fat, 12 g % of daily cal: 7%
Carbohydrate, 260 g % of daily cal: 65%
Protein, 74 g % of daily cal: 19%
Fiber, 27 g
Cholesterol, 99 mg
Calcium, 1257 mg
Sodium, 1225 mg

233

the**Anti-Aging Fitness**
PRESCRIPTION

Activity Map

Low Protein And Hair Loss

An article in the journal *Clinical and Experimental Dermatology* discusses the fact that protein and calorie deficient diets, low nutrient diets or other abnormal eating habits may lead to hair loss. So forget the fancy shampoos and focus on good nutrition.

Your Bodyweight:_____

From Z and Tracy: Time for your Walter Huston dance! Remember when Huston's character does the wacky treasure hunter's dance after they discover a ton of gold in the 1948 movie, *The Treasure of the Sierra Madre*. You didn't see that one? All we have to say is check it out. It has Humphrey Bogart as the lead! Need we say more.

Aerobic Training Exercises

Always start your aerobic activity slowly and gradually progress to your target intensity. Choose one the following aerobic activities and do it for 30 to 40 minutes at an OMNI RPE of 5 to 6.

- Walking (outdoor or indoor)
- Biking (outdoor or indoor)
- Pool walking or exercises or swimming
- Dancing (such as salsa)
- Sports (such as tennis)

Stretching Exercises

Perform all of the following stretching exercises for 2 sets of 15 to 30 seconds.

- Wrist stretch
- Neck stretches
- Hands behind back stretch
- Hands behind head stretch
- Yawn stretch
- Look over the shoulder stretch
- Calf stretch
- Hip flexor stretch
- Hamstring stretch
- Quadriceps stretch
- Inner hip stretch
- Outer hip stretch

Relaxation

Finish your exercise program by lying down and doing the slow relaxation breathing technique for 1 to 5 minutes. You can also perform Tai Chi or Qi Gong as your cool down.

Did You Know That...

The body has approximately 600 total muscles, of which 430 muscles are used for voluntary movement. The body was clearly designed for movement, so get off your couch and take your dog Sparky for a walk!

234

Nutrition Diary

Try Yoga

Yoga is a system of traditional Hindu beliefs, rituals, and activities that is thought to have originated around 3000 B.C. In the Western world, we are most familiar with the physical postures and coordinated diaphragmatic breathing of yoga but yoga also involves meditation and other spiritual practices. Yoga helps to improve flexibility, strength, and balance and also promotes relaxation. There are many types of yoga, including Ashtanga, Kundalini, Iyengar, Bikram, and restorative. Contact a local yoga studio and take a few classes to see if this is a method you want to explore further.

Breakfast

What I ate _____

_____

What I was doing while I ate

_____

Hunger level: **1**   **2**   **3**   **4**   **5**
                Full   Starving

Lunch

What I ate _____

_____

What I was doing while I ate

_____

Hunger level: **1**   **2**   **3**   **4**   **5**
                Full   Starving

Dinner

What I ate _____

_____

What I was doing while I ate

_____

Hunger level: **1**   **2**   **3**   **4**   **5**
                Full   Starving

Snack (if desired)

What I ate _____

_____

What I was doing while I ate

_____

Hunger level: **1**   **2**   **3**   **4**   **5**
                Full   Starving

Suggested Menu

Breakfast
Have 1 serving of Pizza with Roasted Vegetables leftover from Day 34. Serve with 1 red apple. Serve with 1 stick string cheese and 1½ cups fat-free milk.

Lunch
Have 1 serving of the Asian Mixed Green Salad with persimmons instead of mandarin oranges. (Make whole recipe, save ½ for Day 36.)

Snack
Have 1 Pria bar. Serve with 1 cup fat-free milk. Serve with 1 kiwi.

Dinner
Have 1 serving of Tasty Turkey Burger. (Make ½ of recipe, save for Day 36.) Serve topped with 2 tbsp ketchup and mustard if desired. Serve with 1 serving of Baked Acorn Squash leftover from Day 34.

Daily Calorie total: 1598
Fat, 32 g % of daily cal: 18%
Saturated Fat, 9 g % of daily cal: 6%
Carbohydrate, 241 g % of daily cal: 60%
Protein, 100 g % of daily cal: 25%
Fiber, 25 g
Cholesterol, 150 mg
Calcium, 1227 mg
Sodium, 2276 mg

235

Activity Map

Building Your Home Gym

So you want to exercise in your home. Great! The following are some suggestions:

• **Your Living Room:** Place your dumbbells and elastic bands under your couch and pull them out when you watch television.

• **Your Garage:** Convert a part of your garage into a gym.

• **Your Basement:** Convert a section of your basement into a gym and game room.

• **Your Patio/Porch:** Section off a portion of your patio / porch to allow you to ride a stationary or do mat exercises and stretching outdoors in the fresh air.

From Z and Tracy: From this point on it's going to be a straightforward program. This week you'll do three strength training workouts and four aerobic. The next week you'll do five aerobic (like last week) and two strength workouts. Just keep alternating each week with the aerobic and strength workouts so that you get optimal recovery and progression in both areas.

Aerobic Training Exercises

Always start your aerobic activity slowly and gradually progress to your target intensity. Choose one the following aerobic activities and do it for 30 to 45 minutes at an OMNI RPE of 6 to 7.

• Walking (outdoor or indoor)
• Biking (outdoor or indoor)
• Pool walking or exercises or swimming

• Dancing (such as salsa)
• Sports (such as tennis)

Stretching Exercises

Perform all of the following stretching exercises for 2 to 3 sets of 15 to 30 seconds.

• Wrist stretch
• Neck stretches
• Hands behind back stretch
• Hands behind head stretch
• Yawn stretch
• Look over the shoulder stretch

• Calf stretch
• Hip flexor stretch
• Hamstring stretch
• Quadriceps stretch
• Inner hip stretch
• Outer hip stretch

Relaxation

Finish your exercise program by lying down and doing the slow relaxation breathing technique for 1 to 5 minutes. You can also perform Tai Chi or Qi Gong as your cool down.

Anti-Aging Hint:

Avoid wearing tight and restrictive clothing which can reduce blood flow and may lead to pain and discomfort.

236

Nutrition Diary

Your Digestive Engine

Constipation is a common problem in Western countries and can be responsible for a variety medical conditions (such as headaches). You can help prevent constipation by staying active, drinking plenty of fluids, eating a balanced diet which includes vegetables and fruits and finally keeping stress levels under control. Make sure you respond when nature calls and avoid the urge to "hold it" for long periods. Also don't hurry to finish the elimination process when on the toilet.

So for good health, establish a regular pattern of being on the toilet in the morning. Make sure you exercise, since there is some scientific evidence that suggests that low intensity physical activity may have protective effects on the gastrointestinal tract. Finally, if you have chronic constipation (or diarrhea, for that matter), go see your doctor.

Breakfast

What I ate _____

_____

What I was doing while I ate

_____

Hunger level: **1**   **2**   **3**   **4**   **5**
               Full   Starving

Lunch

What I ate _____

_____

What I was doing while I ate

_____

Hunger level: **1**   **2**   **3**   **4**   **5**
               Full   Starving

Dinner

What I ate _____

_____

What I was doing while I ate

_____

Hunger level: **1**   **2**   **3**   **4**   **5**
               Full   Starving

Snack (if desired)

What I ate _____

_____

What I was doing while I ate

_____

Hunger level: **1**   **2**   **3**   **4**   **5**
               Full   Starving

Suggested Menu

Breakfast
Have 1 serving Filo Ricotta Crisps. (Make whole recipe, save remainder for Day 38.) Serve with 1 sliced orange and 1 cup fat-free milk.

Lunch
Split and toast 1 whole wheat hamburger bun, add one Tasty Turkey Burger leftover from Day 35. Top with 2 tbsp ketchup and mustard if desired, sliced tomato and ½ cup baby spinach leaves. Serve with 1 cup fat-free milk.

Snack
Have 1 serving Pizza with Roasted Vegetables from Day 34. Serve with 1 kiwi.

Dinner
Have 1 serving of Asian Mixed Green Salad leftover from Day 35. For dessert, have 4 Hershey's kisses.

Daily Calorie total: 1646
Fat, 40 g % of daily cal: 22%
Saturated Fat, 17 g % of daily cal: 9%
Carbohydrate, 218 g % of daily cal: 53%
Protein, 118 g % of daily cal: 29%
Fiber, 25 g
Cholesterol, 217 mg
Calcium, 1422 mg
Sodium, 2985 mg

237

theAnti-Aging Fitness
PRESCRIPTION

Activity Map

Create Your Home Sports Center

• Put up a basketball rim or a badminton net in your yard.

• Create a section in your backyard for horseshoes.

• Create a section in your backyard for lawn bowling.

• Get a table tennis (ping pong) table for your basement.

• Install a small enclosed fitness pool in your backyard.

• Get two small goals and play backyard soccer.

From Z and Tracy: Your strength workout increases to 2 to 3 sets and you can add some resistance to make the workout harder. Also don't forget that we added an extra set to your balance exercises.

Warm Up Exercises

Perform all of the following warm up exercises for 1 set of 10 reps for each exercise.

• March in place
• Shake, rattle and roll
• Trunk rotations
• Lower back cat / camel

• Heel sits with arms in front
• Heel sits with arms to side
• Hip windshield wiper

Strength Training Exercises

Perform all of the following muscle building and toning exercises for 2 to 3 sets of 8 to 12 reps at an OMNI RPE of 6 to 7.

• Wall ball squats
• Heel raises
• Partial step-ups
• Elastic pull to chest
• Elastic outward rotation
• Dumbbell overhead press

• Modified pushups
• Elastic triceps pushdown
• Dumbbell biceps curl
• Side bridging
• Exercise ball abdominal curls
• Pelvic floor contract, hold, release

Balance Exercises

Perform both balance exercises for 2 to 3 sets of 30 to 60 seconds.

• Very slow motion balancing and walking in place

• Dancer's balance

Stretching Exercises

Perform all of the following stretching exercises for 2 to 3 sets of 15 to 30 seconds.

• Wrist stretch
• Neck stretches
• Hands behind back stretch
• Hands behind head stretch
• Yawn stretch
• Look over the shoulder stretch

• Calf stretch
• Hip flexor stretch
• Hamstring stretch
• Quadriceps stretch
• Inner hip stretch
• Outer hip stretch

Relaxation

Finish your exercise program by lying down and doing the slow relaxation breathing technique for 1 to 5 minutes. You can also perform Tai Chi or Qi Gong as your cool down.

Nutrition Diary

Go Nuts!

Nuts have a pretty bad reputation because they are high in fat. Studies show that people who have nuts as a part of their day report feeling fuller and better able to adhere to a set number of calories. Nuts have unsaturated fats, which are helpful for absorption of vitamins A, D, E, and K; are high in magnesium, which may help reduce the risk for high blood pressure; and contain selenium, which may protect against prostate and colon cancers.

Have a serving of nuts every day.

Soy Nuts: One third cup or 180 nuts

Pistachios: ½ cup with shells or 47 nuts

Almonds: ¼ cup or 23 nuts

Walnut Halves, Pecan Halves or Cashews: ¼ cup or 13 to 18 nuts

Peanuts: ¼ cup or 30 peanuts

Pecan Halves: ¼ cup or 16 nuts

Walnut Halves: ¼ cup without shells or 13 nuts

Breakfast

What I ate _____

_____

What I was doing while I ate

_____

Hunger level: **1**   **2**   **3**   **4**   **5**
            Full   Starving

Lunch

What I ate _____

_____

What I was doing while I ate

_____

Hunger level: **1**   **2**   **3**   **4**   **5**
            Full   Starving

Dinner

What I ate _____

_____

What I was doing while I ate

_____

Hunger level: **1**   **2**   **3**   **4**   **5**
            Full   Starving

Snack (if desired)

What I ate _____

_____

What I was doing while I ate

_____

Hunger level: **1**   **2**   **3**   **4**   **5**
            Full   Starving

Suggested Menu

Breakfast
Have 1 Yogurt Bowl. Serve with 1 cup fat-free milk.

Lunch
Have 1 serving Fast Falafel. Serve 1 one cup fresh black-berries.

Snack
Serve ⅛ cup pistachios with 1 cup cantaloupe cubes.

Dinner
Have 1 serving of Shrimp Caesar Salad. (Make whole recipe, save ½ for Day 38.) For dessert, have 1 low fat ice cream sandwich.

Daily Calorie total: 1570
Fat, 43 g % of daily cal: 25%
Saturated Fat, 8 g % of daily cal: 5%
Carbohydrate, 220 g % of daily cal: 56%
Protein, 97 g % of daily cal: 25%
Fiber, 37 g
Cholesterol, 165 mg
Calcium, 1350 mg
Sodium, 2915 mg

239

the **Anti-Aging Fitness**
PRESCRIPTION

Activity Map

Home Circuit Training

Circuit training is a training method which involves moving from one exercise to the other with varying amounts of rest or stretching in between.

The following is a sample circuit-training routine:

Start with gentle calisthenics as a warm up → Walk 5 minutes → Stop and do 10 to 15 push-ups on a wall → Walk 5 minutes → Stop and do 10 to 15 partial squats → Walk 5 minutes → Stop and do 10 to 15 calf raises → Walk 5 minutes → Stop and do 10 to 15 push-ups on a wall → Walk 5 minutes → Stop and do 10 to 15 partial squats → Walk 5 minutes → End with gentle stretching exercises.

Anti-Aging Hint:

Think safety first. Wear your seatbelts, drive carefully, don't smoke and drink alcohol only in moderation (if at all).

Aerobic Training Exercises

Always start your aerobic activity slowly and gradually progress to your target intensity. Choose one the following aerobic activities and do it for 30 to 45 minutes at an OMNI RPE of 6 to 7.

- Walking (outdoor or indoor)
- Biking (outdoor or indoor)
- Pool walking or exercises or swimming
- Dancing (such as salsa)
- Sports (such as tennis)

Stretching Exercises

Perform all of the following stretching exercises for 2 to 3 sets of 15 to 30 seconds.

- Wrist stretch
- Neck stretches
- Hands behind back stretch
- Hands behind head stretch
- Yawn stretch
- Look over the shoulder stretch
- Calf stretch
- Hip flexor stretch
- Hamstring stretch
- Quadriceps stretch
- Inner hip stretch
- Outer hip stretch

Relaxation

Finish your exercise program by lying down and doing the slow relaxation breathing technique for 1 to 5 minutes. You can also perform Tai Chi or Qi Gong as your cool down.

240

Nutrition Diary

Mighty Magnesium

Magnesium helps maintain normal muscle and nerve function, keeps heart rhythm steady, supports a healthy immune system and keeps bones strong. It also helps regulate blood sugar levels, promotes normal blood pressure, and is involved in energy metabolism and protein synthesis. For adults 31 years old and up, men need 420 mg per day and women need 320 mg. Here are some key foods rich in magnesium:

Halibut, 3 ounces, 90 mg

Almonds, 24 nuts or 1 ounce, 80 mg

Cashews, 18 nuts or 1 ounce, 75 mg

Spinach, ½ cup cooked, 75 mg

Peanut butter, 2 tablespoons, 50 mg

Yogurt, 1 cup plain, 45 mg

Breakfast

What I ate _____

_____

What I was doing while I ate

_____

Hunger level:　**1**　　**2**　　**3**　　**4**　　**5**
　　　　　　　Full　　　　　　　Starving

Lunch

What I ate _____

_____

What I was doing while I ate

_____

Hunger level:　**1**　　**2**　　**3**　　**4**　　**5**
　　　　　　　Full　　　　　　　Starving

Dinner

What I ate _____

_____

What I was doing while I ate

_____

Hunger level:　**1**　　**2**　　**3**　　**4**　　**5**
　　　　　　　Full　　　　　　　Starving

Snack (if desired)

What I ate _____

_____

What I was doing while I ate

_____

Hunger level:　**1**　　**2**　　**3**　　**4**　　**5**
　　　　　　　Full　　　　　　　Starving

Suggested Menu

Breakfast
Make whole recipe Feta Broccoli Fritatta. Have 1 serving, and save 1 serving for Day 39. Serve with 1 tangelo and 1 cup low fat plain yogurt.

Lunch
Have 1 serving of Shrimp Caesar Salad leftover from Day 37. Serve with one green pear.

Snack
Have 1 serving Filo Ricotta Crisps leftover from Day 35.

Dinner
Have 1 serving Sweet and Sour Apricot Salsa Chicken. Make whole recipe, save ½ for Day 39. For dessert, make 1 serving Pudding Parfait.

Daily Calorie total: 1620
Fat, 46 g % of daily cal: 26%
Saturated Fat, 20 g % of daily cal: 11%
Carbohydrate, 191 g % of daily cal: 47%
Protein, 123 g % of daily cal: 30%
Fiber, 26 g
Cholesterol, 517 mg
Calcium, 1633 mg
Sodium, 3072 mg

241

Activity Map

Home Interval Training

Interval training is a training method where periods of exercise (higher-intensity interval, such as fast walking) are alternated with periods of relief (lower-intensity interval, such as slow walking).

An example of a simple interval training program would be to walk fast for 2 minutes and then walk slow for 6 minutes. This fast-walk/slow-walk cycle can be repeated for 15 to 30 minutes.

Aerobic Training Exercises

Always start your aerobic activity slowly and gradually progress to your target intensity. Choose one the following aerobic activities and do it for 30 to 45 minutes at an OMNI RPE of 6 to 7.

- Walking (outdoor or indoor)
- Biking (outdoor or indoor)
- Pool walking or exercises or swimming
- Dancing (such as salsa)
- Sports (such as tennis)

Stretching Exercises

Perform all of the following stretching exercises for 2 to 3 sets of 15 to 30 seconds.

- Wrist stretch
- Neck stretches
- Hands behind back stretch
- Hands behind head stretch
- Yawn stretch
- Look over the shoulder stretch
- Calf stretch
- Hip flexor stretch
- Hamstring stretch
- Quadriceps stretch
- Inner hip stretch
- Outer hip stretch

Relaxation

Finish your exercise program by lying down and doing the slow relaxation breathing technique for 1 to 5 minutes. You can also perform Tai Chi or Qi Gong as your cool down.

Nutrition Diary

Hyponatremia – Are You At Risk?

Hyponatremia, a dangerously low sodium level in your blood, can lead to diminished brain, heart and muscle function and eventually death. It's all the buzz right now, but are you really at risk? Symptoms of hyponatremia include nausea, muscle cramps, disorientation, slurred speech, confusion.

Unless you're an endurance athlete, your risk for hyponatremia is minimal, and the benefit from keeping your diet low in sodium far outweighs any danger from low sodium intake. People at risk for hyponatremia include those who are exercising an hour or more, drinking a gallon or more of water and not replacing sodium lost through sweating. Instead, prepare for an event by having a snack or meal with 1,000 mg or more of sodium and hydrate yourself with 16 ounces of water an hour before the event. During events lasting more than one hour, drink electrolyte replacement drinks such as Gatorade®.

Breakfast

What I ate _____

_____

What I was doing while I ate

_____

Hunger level: **1   2   3   4   5**
              Full   Starving

Lunch

What I ate _____

_____

What I was doing while I ate

_____

Hunger level: **1   2   3   4   5**
              Full   Starving

Dinner

What I ate _____

_____

What I was doing while I ate

_____

Hunger level: **1   2   3   4   5**
              Full   Starving

Snack (if desired)

What I ate _____

_____

What I was doing while I ate

_____

Hunger level: **1   2   3   4   5**
              Full   Starving

Suggested Menu

Breakfast
Have 1 serving of Feta Broccoli Fritatta leftover from Day 38. Serve with 1 cup fat-free milk and 2 fresh apricots.

Lunch
Have 1 serving Sweet and Sour Apricot Salsa Chicken leftover from Day 38. Serve with 1 serving Tasty Greens, use kale. Make whole recipe; save ½ for Day 40.

Snack
Have 1 serving of Festival of Fruit Salad. (Make ½ of recipe; save 1 serving for Day 40.) Serve with 1 cup low fat vanilla yogurt.

Dinner
Have 1 serving Glazed Pork and Apples. For dessert, have 1 lowfat ice cream sandwich.

Daily Calorie total: 1587
Fat, 35 g % of daily cal: 20%
Saturated Fat, 10 g % of daily cal: 6%
Carbohydrate, 218 g % of daily cal: 55%
Protein, 103 g % of daily cal: 26%
Fiber, 26 g
Cholesterol, 356 mg
Calcium, 1243 mg
Sodium, 1881 mg

243

the**Anti-Aging Fitness**
PRESCRIPTION

Activity Map

Try Cross Training

Cross training is a training method where exercises (such as treadmill, recumbent bike, upper body bike, or elliptical trainer) or activities (such as walking, outdoor bicycling, swimming, circuit weight training or calisthenics) are varied in either a single workout or during the week. The advantage of cross training is that by varying the activities, you reduce the stress and strain on your body, prevent overtraining, allow for better recovery, and improve your fitness. One example of a simple cross-training program would be to walk for 30 minutes on Monday, do 30 minutes of outdoor or indoor bicycling on Wednesday and 30 minutes of swimming on Friday. Just be creative and design your own program.

Warm Up Exercises

Always start your aerobic activity slowly and gradually progress to your target intensity. Choose one of the following aerobic activities and do it for 10 to 15 minutes at an OMNI RPE of 1 to 2:

- March in place
- Shake, rattle and roll
- Trunk rotations
- Lower back cat / camel
- Heel sits with arms in front
- Heel sits with arms to side
- Hip windshield wiper

Strength Training Exercises

Perform all of the following muscle building and toning exercises for 2 to 3 sets of 8 to 12 reps at an OMNI RPE of 6 to 7.

- Wall ball squats
- Heel raises
- Partial step-ups
- Elastic pull to chest
- Elastic outward rotation
- Dumbbell overhead press
- Modified pushups
- Elastic triceps pushdown
- Dumbbell biceps curl
- Side bridging
- Exercise ball abdominal curls
- Pelvic floor contract, hold, release

Balance Exercises

Perform both balance exercises for 2 to 3 sets of 30 to 60 seconds.

- Very slow motion balancing and walking in place
- Dancer's balance

Stretching Exercises

Perform all of the following stretching exercises for 2 to 3 sets of 15 to 30 seconds.

- Wrist stretch
- Neck stretches
- Hands behind back stretch
- Hands behind head stretch
- Yawn stretch
- Look over the shoulder stretch
- Calf stretch
- Hip flexor stretch
- Hamstring stretch
- Quadriceps stretch
- Inner hip stretch
- Outer hip stretch

Relaxation

Finish your exercise program by lying down and doing the slow relaxation breathing technique for 1 to 5 minutes. You can also perform Tai Chi or Qi Gong as your cool down.

Nutrition Diary

Sodium Sense

Controlling blood pressure is critical for reducing our risk for heart attack and stroke. Processed foods account for the majority of the sodium we consume.

• Use no salt added canned foods and low sodium soup.

• For spaghetti sauce, choose 350 mg sodium or less per half cup serving.

• Barbeque sauce, soy sauce and salad dressing can be very high in sodium. Choose the lower sodium versions whenever possible.

• Rinse canned foods such as beans, tuna in a colander under cold, running water for 2 to 3 minutes to remove some of the sodium.

Breakfast

What I ate _____

_____

What I was doing while I ate

_____

Hunger level: **1**   **2**   **3**   **4**   **5**
        Full   Starving

Lunch

What I ate _____

_____

What I was doing while I ate

_____

Hunger level: **1**   **2**   **3**   **4**   **5**
        Full   Starving

Dinner

What I ate _____

_____

What I was doing while I ate

_____

Hunger level: **1**   **2**   **3**   **4**   **5**
        Full   Starving

Snack (if desired)

What I ate _____

_____

What I was doing while I ate

_____

Hunger level: **1**   **2**   **3**   **4**   **5**
        Full   Starving

Suggested Menu

Breakfast

Have 1 serving of the Festival of Fruit Salad leftover from Day 39. Serve fruit salad over 1 cup 1% cottage cheese.

Lunch

Have one 6" whole wheat pita bread toasted spread with 2 tbsp hummus and filled with ½ cup canned black beans, ½ cup canned yellow corn, and 5 halved grape tomatoes. Serve with 1 portion of Tasty Greens leftover from Day 39.

Snack

Have 1 Pria bar with 1 cup honeydew cubes and 1 slice soy cheese.

Dinner

Have 1 serving Chicken Curry. (Make whole recipe, save 1 serving for Day 41.) For dessert, have 4 Hershey's kisses.

Daily Calorie total: 1558
Fat, 38 g % of daily cal: 22%
Saturated Fat, 12 g % of daily cal: 7%
Carbohydrate, 194 g % of daily cal: 50%
Protein, 99 g % of daily cal: 25%
Fiber, 33 g
Cholesterol, 80 mg
Calcium, 1350 mg
Sodium, 2678 mg

the**Anti-Aging Fitness**
PRESCRIPTION

Activity Map

Fitness In Your Community

- Go to a rink for ice skating or roller skating.
- Go bowling.
- Go to the driving range and hit a bucket of balls.
- Go to the batting cage and swing a bat at a few balls.

Aerobic Training Exercises

Always start your aerobic activity slowly and gradually progress to your target intensity. Choose one the following aerobic activities and do it for 30 to 45 minutes at an OMNI RPE of 6 to 7.

- Walking (outdoor or indoor)
- Biking (outdoor or indoor)
- Pool walking or exercises or swimming
- Dancing (such as salsa)
- Sports (such as tennis)

Stretching Exercises

Perform all of the following stretching exercises for 2 to 3 sets of 15 to 30 seconds.

- Wrist stretch
- Neck stretches
- Hands behind back stretch
- Hands behind head stretch
- Yawn stretch
- Look over the shoulder stretch
- Calf stretch
- Hip flexor stretch
- Hamstring stretch
- Quadriceps stretch
- Inner hip stretch
- Outer hip stretch

Relaxation

Finish your exercise program by lying down and doing the slow relaxation breathing technique for 1 to 5 minutes. You can also perform Tai Chi or Qi Gong as your cool down.

246

Nutrition Diary

Potassium

We've established the fact that as you age, your risk of bone loss, stroke, and high blood pressure increase. Potassium is critical to managing all three and it's plentiful in your anti-aging plan. Here is a list of foods high in potassium; the amount is listed in milligrams (mg):

Potato, ½ cup, 940 mg

Sweet Potato, ½ cup, 540 mg

Banana, 490 mg

Halibut, 3 ounces cooked, 490 mg

Spinach, 420 mg

Cantaloupe, ¼ melon, 370 mg

People with kidney disease, diabetes and people using blood pressure medication and other drugs should first ask their doctor before increasing their intake of potassium from foods.

Breakfast

What I ate _____

_____

What I was doing while I ate

_____

Hunger level: **1   2   3   4   5**
        Full   Starving

Lunch

What I ate _____

_____

What I was doing while I ate

_____

Hunger level: **1   2   3   4   5**
        Full   Starving

Dinner

What I ate _____

_____

What I was doing while I ate

_____

Hunger level: **1   2   3   4   5**
        Full   Starving

Snack (if desired)

What I ate _____

_____

What I was doing while I ate

_____

Hunger level: **1   2   3   4   5**
        Full   Starving

Suggested Menu

Breakfast
Have 1 serving Tropical Cereal. Serve with 1 cup fat-free milk and 1 pomegranate.

Lunch
Have 1 serving Chicken Curry leftover from Day 40.

Snack
Have 10 baby carrots, dip in 2 tbsp light salad dressing.

Dinner
Have 1 serving Pasta Primavera. (Make whole recipe, save ½ for Day 42.) For dessert, have 1 regular fudgesicle.

Daily Calorie total: 1616
Fat, 36 g % of daily cal: 20%
Saturated Fat, 14 g % of daily cal: 8%
Carbohydrate, 243 g % of daily cal: 60%
Protein, 86 g % of daily cal: 21%
Fiber, 33 g
Cholesterol, 145 mg
Calcium, 1541 mg
Sodium, 1693 mg

the **Anti-Aging Fitness**
PRESCRIPTION

Activity Map

Saving Your Hearing With Earplugs

There are two ways the ear can be damaged by noise. One way is from exposure to high-level, short-duration noise exposures exceeding 140 decibels from events, such as a fire-cracker or toy cap gun going off near the ear or from a shotgun, high-powered rifle or pistol. The second is noise-induced hearing loss which is a type of hearing loss which develops slowly over years and is caused by any exposure to noise (including music) regularly exceeding a daily average of 90 decibels from events, such as listening to loud music, going to a rock concert, going to a club that plays loud music, using machinery (such as lawn mowers or vacuum cleaners) or riding a motorcycle. So wear appropriate hearing protection to save your hearing.

Your Bodyweight:_____

From Z and Tracy: Six weeks down. Now we're starting to cruise.

Warm Up Exercises

Perform all of the following warm up exercises for 1 set of 10 reps for each exercise.

- March in place
- Shake, rattle and roll
- Trunk rotations
- Lower back cat / camel
- Heel sits with arms in front
- Heel sits with arms to side
- Hip windshield wiper

Strength Training Exercises

Perform all of the following muscle building and toning exercises for 2 to 3 sets of 8 to 12 reps at an OMNI RPE of 6 to 7.

- Wall ball squats
- Heel raises
- Partial step-ups
- Elastic pull to chest
- Elastic outward rotation
- Dumbbell overhead press
- Modified pushups
- Elastic triceps pushdown
- Dumbbell biceps curl
- Side bridging
- Exercise ball abdominal curls
- Pelvic floor contract, hold, release

Balance Exercises

Perform both balance exercises for 2 to 3 sets of 30 to 60 seconds.

- Very slow motion balancing and walking in place
- Dancer's balance

Stretching Exercises

Perform all of the following stretching exercises for 2 to 3 sets of 15 to 30 seconds.

- Wrist stretch
- Neck stretches
- Hands behind back stretch
- Hands behind head stretch
- Yawn stretch
- Look over the shoulder stretch
- Calf stretch
- Hip flexor stretch
- Hamstring stretch
- Quadriceps stretch
- Inner hip stretch
- Outer hip stretch

Relaxation

Finish your exercise program by lying down and doing the slow relaxation breathing technique for 1 to 5 minutes. You can also perform Tai Chi or Qi Gong as your cool down.

Nutrition Diary

Challenge Yourself – Try Pilates

Pilates is a form of body work that uses controlled movements and poses to improve strength, flexibility, balance and mental concentration. Joseph H. Pilates is the creator of this system. In the 1920's he developed his 34 core exercises that were to be performed on a mat without any specialized equipment. Later he developed many original exercise machines that are used today for fitness. Contact a local Pilates studio and take a few lessons to see if this is a method you want to further explore.

Breakfast

What I ate _____

_____

What I was doing while I ate

_____

Hunger level: **1**   **2**   **3**   **4**   **5**
              Full   Starving

Lunch

What I ate _____

_____

What I was doing while I ate

_____

Hunger level: **1**   **2**   **3**   **4**   **5**
              Full   Starving

Dinner

What I ate _____

_____

What I was doing while I ate

_____

Hunger level: **1**   **2**   **3**   **4**   **5**
              Full   Starving

Snack (if desired)

What I ate _____

_____

What I was doing while I ate

_____

Hunger level: **1**   **2**   **3**   **4**   **5**
              Full   Starving

Suggested Menu

Breakfast

Have 1 packet regular flavor instant oatmeal made with ½ cup fat-free milk and topped with 1 tbsp chopped walnuts.

Lunch

Have 1 serving Pasta Primavera leftover from Day 41.

Snack

Have ¾ cup low fat vanilla yogurt (save remaining ¼ cup for Day 43) and ½ sliced mango (save the other half for Day 43).

Dinner

Have 1 serving Crab Cakes. (Make whole recipe; save ½ for Day 43.) Serve with a side salad made with 2 cups romaine lettuce topped with 1 cup halved red grapes, 1 chopped green apple and 2 tbsp raspberry vinaigrette salad dressing. For dessert, have ½ cup of ice cream.

Daily Calorie total: 1626
Fat, 61 g % of daily cal: 34%
Saturated Fat, 16 g % of daily cal: 9%
Carbohydrate, 214 g % of daily cal: 53%
Protein, 79 g % of daily cal: 19%
Fiber, 22 g
Cholesterol, 320 mg
Calcium, 1238 mg
Sodium, 1914 mg

249

Activity Map

Soothing Sounds For Your Mind And Body

Various sounds can have a soothing effect on the mind and body. Music and pleasant sounds such as the following can reduce anxiety, stress and pain.

• Rustling leaves.

• Songbirds.

• Flowing water at a stream or river.

• Ocean or lake water breaking at a beach.

• Light rain.

• Wind chimes.

• Music such as Mozart.

• Singing.

• Whistling.

• Laughter on TV.

From Z and Tracy: You're now entering our maintenance phase. It doesn't mean that you can't progress anymore but you have the option of putting things into cruise control and maintaining the progress that you've made. At another time, say 8 to 12 weeks later, you can try another building phase if you wish. This delay in pushing yourself can allow your body to adjust to the past 8 weeks of hard work you put into the program. From here on out we're keeping your cardio at 30 to 45 minutes, strength program at 2 to 3 sets of 8 to 15 reps, stretching program at 1 to 3 sets of 15 to 30 seconds and finally, your balance exercises at 1 to 3 sets of 30 to 60 seconds .

Aerobic Training Exercises

Always start your aerobic activity slowly and gradually progress to your target intensity. Choose one the following aerobic activities and do it for 30 to 45 minutes at an OMNI RPE of 5 to 7.

• Walking (outdoor or indoor)
• Biking (outdoor or indoor)
• Pool walking or exercises or swimming
• Dancing (such as salsa)
• Sports (such as tennis)

Stretching Exercises

Perform all of the following stretching exercises for 1 to 3 sets of 15 to 30 seconds.

• Wrist stretch
• Neck stretches
• Hands behind back stretch
• Hands behind head stretch
• Yawn stretch
• Look over the shoulder stretch
• Calf stretch
• Hip flexor stretch
• Hamstring stretch
• Quadriceps stretch
• Inner hip stretch
• Outer hip stretch

Relaxation

Finish your exercise program by lying down and doing the slow relaxation breathing technique for 1 to 5 minutes. You can also perform Tai Chi or Qi Gong as your cool down.

Nutrition Diary

Deciphering Health Information

Carrots are bad for diabetics. A high saturated fat diet shows a reduced risk of stroke. With all of these news stories and tips online and on the air, it can be frustrating for the educated listener to decide how to handle health information. Look at the source of the study, and determine if the publication is a peer-reviewed journal. This is generally an indication of good quality writing.

Rarely will a researcher make recommendations based on the results of one study. Check out the long-term studies involving thousands of people such as NHANES (National Health and Nutrition Examination Survey), which examines trends in major chronic diseases and the relationship of observed risk factors, such as diet, to those diseases.

If you hear a piece of information, do some research to find out the source of the study. Go to the website www.ncbi.nlm.nih.gov and then go to PubMed to search specific topics.

Breakfast

What I ate _____

_____

What I was doing while I ate

_____

Hunger level: **1   2   3   4   5**
        Full   Starving

Lunch

What I ate _____

_____

What I was doing while I ate

_____

Hunger level: **1   2   3   4   5**
        Full   Starving

Dinner

What I ate _____

_____

What I was doing while I ate

_____

Hunger level: **1   2   3   4   5**
        Full   Starving

Snack (if desired)

What I ate _____

_____

What I was doing while I ate

_____

Hunger level: **1   2   3   4   5**
        Full   Starving

Suggested Menu

Breakfast
Have 1 serving Filo Ricotta Crisps. (Make whole recipe; ½ for Day 44.) Serve with ½ sliced mango topped with ½ cup low fat vanilla yogurt from Day 42.

Lunch
Have 1 serving Crab Cakes leftover from Day 42. Serve with ½ grapefruit, save ½ for snack on Day 44.

Snack
Have 1 serving Roasted Chickpeas. (Make whole recipe; save ½ for Day 44.) Serve with 1 plum.

Dinner
Have 1 serving Shrimp Caesar Salad. (Make whole recipe; save ½ for Day 44.) For dessert have 1 regular fudgesicle.

Daily Calorie total: 1642
Fat, 57 g %of daily cal: 31%
Saturated Fat, 18 g %of daily cal: 10%
Carbohydrate, 189 g %of daily cal: 46%
Protein, 109 g %of daily cal: 27%
Fiber, 26 g
Cholesterol, 467 mg
Calcium, 1395 mg
Sodium, 2840 mg

Activity Map

Reduce Stress While You Drive

The following are tips to help you enjoy your ride:

• Leave early for an appointment.

• Play relaxing music.

• Keep the car temperature comfortable.

• Use your car air filter to keep the air fresh.

• Loosen up your clothes.

• Do minimal lane changes.

• Don't multi-task by talking on the cell phone.

• Don't put your hands on top of the steering wheel or grip tightly.

• Keep a healthy snack nearby.

• Keep separation between you and the car in front of you.

• Ride with a friend.

• Live close to work.

Warm Up Exercises

Perform all of the following warm up exercises for 1 set of 10 reps for each exercise.

• March in place
• Shake, rattle and roll
• Trunk rotations
• Lower back cat / camel

• Heel sits with arms in front
• Heel sits with arms to side
• Hip windshield wiper

Strength Training Exercises

Perform all of the following muscle building and toning exercises for 2 to 3 sets of 8 to 15 reps at an OMNI RPE of 5 to 7.

• Wall ball squats
• Heel raises
• Partial step-ups
• Elastic pull to chest
• Elastic outward rotation
• Dumbbell overhead press

• Modified pushups
• Elastic triceps pushdown
• Dumbbell biceps curl
• Side bridging
• Exercise ball abdominal curls
• Pelvic floor contract, hold, release

Balance Exercises

Perform both balance exercises for 1 to 3 sets of 30 to 60 seconds.

• Very slow motion balancing and walking in place

• Dancer's balance

Stretching Exercises

Perform all of the following stretching exercises for 1 to 3 sets of 15 to 30 seconds.

• Wrist stretch
• Neck stretches
• Hands behind back stretch
• Hands behind head stretch
• Yawn stretch
• Look over the shoulder stretch

• Calf stretch
• Hip flexor stretch
• Hamstring stretch
• Quadriceps stretch
• Inner hip stretch
• Outer hip stretch

Relaxation

Finish your exercise program by lying down and doing the slow relaxation breathing technique for 1 to 5 minutes. You can also perform Tai Chi or Qi Gong as your cool down.

Nutrition Diary

The Latest Fad?

Different trends surface from time to time and claim to be "the answer." Finally, you breathe a sigh of relief; this diet is going to be the one. You venture forth and learn all the new rules of the latest craze and stock your shelves with foods you wouldn't normally choose.

If you ignore your typical food habits and preferences and attempt a short-term "fix" to get healthy, you'll be right back at square one before you can say Mississippi.

Give yourself permission to keep some of your favorite foods and incorporate these simple healthy recommendations, three meals a day, three servings of calcium-rich foods and three different colored fruits and vegetables every day.

Breakfast

What I ate _____

_____

What I was doing while I ate

_____

Hunger level: **1**   **2**   **3**   **4**   **5**
       Full   Starving

Lunch

What I ate _____

_____

What I was doing while I ate

_____

Hunger level: **1**   **2**   **3**   **4**   **5**
       Full   Starving

Dinner

What I ate _____

_____

What I was doing while I ate

_____

Hunger level: **1**   **2**   **3**   **4**   **5**
       Full   Starving

Snack (if desired)

What I ate _____

_____

What I was doing while I ate

_____

Hunger level: **1**   **2**   **3**   **4**   **5**
       Full   Starving

Suggested Menu

Breakfast
Have 1 Crunchy Banana Pop. (Make whole recipe; save ½ for Day 45.)

Lunch
Have 1 serving Shrimp Caesar Salad leftover from Day 43. Serve with 1 cup cherries.

Snack
Have 1 serving Filo Ricotta Crisps and ½ grapefruit left-over from Day 43.

Dinner
Spread one 8" whole wheat soft tortilla with 2 tbsp hummus, fill with 1 serving of Roasted Chickpeas leftover from Day 43 and 10 halved grape tomatoes and 1 cup baby spinach leaves. For dessert, have 1 frozen fruit juice bar, about 40 calories.

Daily Calorie total: 1617
Fat, 47 g %of daily cal: 26%
Saturated Fat, 15 g %of daily cal: 8%
Carbohydrate, 234 g %of daily cal: 58%
Protein, 88 g %of daily cal: 22%
Fiber, 38 g
Cholesterol, 217 mg
Calcium, 1143 mg
Sodium, 2518 mg

Activity Map

Dance Your Way To Good Health

Dancing is a fun way to get exercise into your routine. Dancing works on your balance, coordination flexibility and endurance. How about:

- Salsa
- Tango
- Square dancing
- Belly dancing
- Ballet
- Ballroom dance
- Swing
- Jazz

Aerobic Training Exercises

Always start your aerobic activity slowly and gradually progress to your target intensity. Choose one the following aerobic activities and do it for 30 to 45 minutes at an OMNI RPE of 5 to 7.

- Walking (outdoor or indoor)
- Biking (outdoor or indoor)
- Pool walking or exercises or swimming
- Dancing (such as salsa)
- Sports (such as tennis)

Stretching Exercises

Perform all of the following stretching exercises for 1 to 3 sets of 15 to 30 seconds.

- Wrist stretch
- Neck stretches
- Hands behind back stretch
- Hands behind head stretch
- Yawn stretch
- Look over the shoulder stretch
- Calf stretch
- Hip flexor stretch
- Hamstring stretch
- Quadriceps stretch
- Inner hip stretch
- Outer hip stretch

Relaxation

Finish your exercise program by lying down and doing the slow relaxation breathing technique for 1 to 5 minutes. You can also perform Tai Chi or Qi Gong as your cool down.

Anti-Aging Hint:

Train your body in a balanced manner, where you focus on the right and left, front and back as well as the upper and lower parts.

254

Nutrition Diary

The Cost of Eating Well

Digest this: the money spent on one bag of chips and one box of cookies could buy ALL of the following; two pounds of apples, one pound of bananas, one pound of carrots, two pounds of potatoes and one pound of peppers. It may seem more expensive to eat healthy foods, but fast food and junk food actually cost more than preparing a meal at home. If you plan well, the cost for a meal prepared at home can be cheap. Choose frozen bags of vegetables, unsweetened frozen bags of fruits, and freeze all bread products and defrost them in the microwave right before serving. And with the exception of lettuce and tomatoes, almost any fresh fruit or vegetable that you buy can be frozen. Take an extra minute to pop a home-cooked meal into the freezer if you're not eating it right away (like our anti-aging recipes).

A little planning for your meals goes a long way towards saving money and making better choices. It's much quicker to defrost a prepared meal from the freezer than it is to wait in line for a fast food meal.

Breakfast

What I ate _____

What I was doing while I ate

Hunger level: **1** **2** **3** **4** **5**
Full   Starving

Lunch

What I ate _____

What I was doing while I ate

Hunger level: **1** **2** **3** **4** **5**
Full   Starving

Dinner

What I ate _____

What I was doing while I ate

Hunger level: **1** **2** **3** **4** **5**
Full   Starving

Snack (if desired)

What I ate _____

What I was doing while I ate

Hunger level: **1** **2** **3** **4** **5**
Full   Starving

Suggested Menu

Breakfast
Have 1 serving Yogurt Bowl Breakfast. Serve with 1 cup fresh or frozen, unsweetened strawberries.

Lunch
Have 1 6" whole wheat sub roll topped with 2 oz sliced chicken breast, 1 cup arugula leaves, ¼ cup red onion, ½ sliced yellow bell pepper spread with Dijon mustard if desired.

Snack
Have 1 serving Crunchy Banana Pop from Day 44. Serve with 1 cup fat-free milk.

Dinner
Have 1 serving Stoplight Pasta. (Make whole recipe; save ½ for Day 46.) For dessert have 1 Frozen Milk Pop.

Daily Calorie total: 1624
Fat, 38 g % of daily cal: 21%
Saturated Fat, 10 g % of daily cal: 6%
Carbohydrate, 254 g % of daily cal: 63%
Protein, 98 g % of daily cal: 24%
Fiber, 37 g
Cholesterol, 103 mg
Calcium, 1707 mg
Sodium, 1894 mg

255

the Anti-Aging Fitness PRESCRIPTION

Activity Map

Martial Arts Fitness

Try martial arts as a form of fitness and to learn how to defend yourself. Consider taking preliminary lessons in several forms to see which one you really enjoy and want to continue long term.

- Aikido
- Hapkido
- Jeet Kune Do
- Judo
- Jujitsu
- Karate
- Kung Fu
- Qi Gong
- Taekwondo
- Tai Chi

Aerobic Training Exercises

Always start your aerobic activity slowly and gradually progress to your target intensity. Choose one the following aerobic activities and do it for 30 to 45 minutes at an OMNI RPE of 5 to 7.

- Walking (outdoor or indoor)
- Biking (outdoor or indoor)
- Pool walking or exercises or swimming
- Dancing (such as salsa)
- Sports (such as tennis)

Stretching Exercises

Perform all of the following stretching exercises for 1 to 3 sets of 15 to 30 seconds.

- Wrist stretches
- Neck stretches
- Hands behind back stretch
- Hands behind head stretch
- Yawn stretch
- Look over the shoulder stretch
- Calf stretch
- Hip flexor stretch
- Hamstring stretch
- Quadriceps stretch
- Inner hip stretch
- Outer hip stretch

Relaxation

Finish your exercise program by lying down and doing the slow relaxation breathing technique for 1 to 5 minutes. You can also perform Tai Chi or Qi Gong as your cool down.

Anti-Aging Hint:

If you want to lose weight, then don't skip meals, don't "supersize," avoid late night eating, and watch your portion sizes on your plate.

256

Nutrition Diary

Filters For Good Health

Commercial filters can help purify the air you breathe and the water that you drink. Air filters in your home or office can help you if you suffer from pollen or other airborne allergens. Water filters on your shower and kitchen sink can help to reduce skin irritation and keep pollutants off of your fruits and vegetables. Studies have shown that plants have the ability to purify various atmospheric pollutants. One study in the *International Journal of Phytoremediation* in 2003 shows promise that the plant, Golden Pothos, has air purification capabilities for atmospheric gasoline.

Breakfast

What I ate _____

_____

What I was doing while I ate

_____

Hunger level: **1**   **2**   **3**   **4**   **5**
                    Full   Starving

Lunch

What I ate _____

_____

What I was doing while I ate

_____

Hunger level: **1**   **2**   **3**   **4**   **5**
                    Full   Starving

Dinner

What I ate _____

_____

What I was doing while I ate

_____

Hunger level: **1**   **2**   **3**   **4**   **5**
                    Full   Starving

Snack (if desired)

What I ate _____

_____

What I was doing while I ate

_____

Hunger level: **1**   **2**   **3**   **4**   **5**
                    Full   Starving

Suggested Menu

Breakfast
Have 1 serving Fluffy Orange Pancakes. (Make whole recipe, save remainder for Days 47, 48, and 49.) Serve with 1 cup fat-free milk and 1 sliced guava.

Lunch
Have 1 serving Stoplight Pasta leftover from Day 45. Serve with 1 cup fresh green beans topped with 1 tbsp balsamic vinaigrette dressing.

Snack
Have 1 cup fresh raspberries mixed with 1 sliced kiwi.

Dinner
Have 1 serving Turkey Empanadas. (Make whole recipe; save ½ for Day 47.) Serve with 1 small baked sweet potato, top with 1 serving Sweet Cream Spread. (Make 2 servings, save 1 serving for Day 47.) For dessert, have 1 regular fudgesicle.

Daily Calorie total: 1601
Fat, 32 g % of daily cal: 18%
Saturated Fat, 12 g % of daily cal: 7%
Carbohydrate, 251 g % of daily cal: 63%
Protein, 96 g % of daily cal: 24%
Fiber, 38 g
Cholesterol, 331 mg
Calcium, 1329 mg
Sodium, 2513 mg

257

the Anti-Aging Fitness
PRESCRIPTION

Activity Map

Try Tennis And Golf

Both tennis and golf are social activities that can be geared for your pace. Both activities involve mental and physical challenges and both activities involve being in peaceful surroundings with fresh air and sunshine. So take some tennis and golf lessons and start having fun.

Anti-Aging Hint:

Plato said "Life must be lived as play." So being active isn't much of a chore if your activity is more a game than a task.

258

Warm Up Exercises

Perform all of the following warm up exercises for 1 set of 10 reps for each exercise.

- March in place
- Shake, rattle and roll
- Trunk rotations
- Lower back cat / camel
- Heel sits with arms in front
- Heel sits with arms to side
- Hip windshield wiper

Strength Training Exercises

Perform all of the following muscle building and toning exercises for 2 to 3 sets of 8 to 15 reps at an OMNI RPE of 5 to 7.

- Wall ball squats
- Heel raises
- Partial step-ups
- Elastic pull to chest
- Elastic outward rotation
- Dumbbell overhead press
- Modified pushups
- Elastic triceps pushdown
- Dumbbell biceps curl
- Side bridging
- Exercise ball abdominal curls
- Pelvic floor contract, hold, release

Balance Exercises

Perform both balance exercises for 1 to 3 sets of 30 to 60 seconds.

- Very slow motion balancing and walking in place
- Dancer's balance

Stretching Exercises

Perform all of the following stretching exercises for 1 to 3 sets of 15 to 30 seconds.

- Wrist stretch
- Neck stretches
- Hands behind back stretch
- Hands behind head stretch
- Yawn stretch
- Look over the shoulder stretch
- Calf stretch
- Hip flexor stretch
- Hamstring stretch
- Quadriceps stretch
- Inner hip stretch
- Outer hip stretch

Relaxation

Finish your exercise program by lying down and doing the slow relaxation breathing technique for 1 to 5 minutes. You can also perform Tai Chi or Qi Gong as your cool down.

Nutrition Diary

How To Protect Your Joints

• Respect pain. The body may be giving you a signal to modify, reduce, or avoid activity for a period of time.

• Avoid staying in one position for a prolonged period of time.

• Use proper body mechanics for lifting, sitting, standing, and bending.

• Avoid awkward positions that cause strain to your joints.

• Find a balance between work (activity) and rest.

• Get adequate sleep at night for proper recovery.

• Get proper nutrition to allow your body to provide energy, repair, and maintenance.

• Exercise to maintain range of motion, strength, and endurance.

Breakfast

What I ate _____

_____

What I was doing while I ate

_____

Hunger level: **1**   **2**   **3**   **4**   **5**
        Full   Starving

Lunch

What I ate _____

_____

What I was doing while I ate

_____

Hunger level: **1**   **2**   **3**   **4**   **5**
        Full   Starving

Dinner

What I ate _____

_____

What I was doing while I ate

_____

Hunger level: **1**   **2**   **3**   **4**   **5**
        Full   Starving

Snack (if desired)

What I ate _____

_____

What I was doing while I ate

_____

Hunger level: **1**   **2**   **3**   **4**   **5**
        Full   Starving

Suggested Menu

Breakfast
Have 2 waffles topped with 1 serving of Sweet Cream Spread leftover from Day 46. Serve with 1 cup fat-free milk and 1 tangelo.

Lunch
Have 1 serving Turkey Empanadas leftover from Day 46. Serve with 1 cup honey-dew cubes.

Snack
Have 1 serving Fluffy Orange Pancakes leftover from Day 45. Serve with 1 cup blueberries.

Dinner
Have 1 serving Lime Peanut Salad. (Make whole recipe; save ½ for Day 48.) For dessert, have 1 Pria bar.

Daily Calorie total: 1629
Fat, 41 g % of daily cal: 23%
Saturated Fat, 10 g % of daily cal: 6%
Carbohydrate, 249 g % of daily cal: 61%
Protein, 85 g % of daily cal: 21%
Fiber, 29 g
Cholesterol, 209 mg
Calcium, 1196 mg
Sodium, 2644 mg

259

Activity Map

Play With Your Kids

Why not try playing with your kids and grandchildren as a part of being active? Movement doesn't always have to be choreographed and regimented exercise in order for it to be effective. Chasing after those little rascals can be quite a workout.

Aerobic Training Exercises

Always start your aerobic activity slowly and gradually progress to your target intensity. Choose one the following aerobic activities and do it for 30 to 45 minutes at an OMNI RPE of 5 to 7.

- Walking (outdoor or indoor)
- Biking (outdoor or indoor)
- Pool walking or exercises or swimming
- Dancing (such as salsa)
- Sports (such as tennis)

Stretching Exercises

Perform all of the following stretching exercises for 1 to 3 sets of 15 to 30 seconds.

- Wrist stretch
- Neck stretches
- Hands behind back stretch
- Hands behind head stretch
- Yawn stretch
- Look over the shoulder stretch
- Calf stretch
- Hip flexor stretch
- Hamstring stretch
- Quadriceps stretch
- Inner hip stretch
- Outer hip stretch

Relaxation

Finish your exercise program by lying down and doing the slow relaxation breathing technique for 1 to 5 minutes. You can also perform Tai Chi or Qi Gong as your cool down.

Nutrition Diary

How To Prevent A Fall

- Use a nightlight for going to the bathroom at night.
- Use non-slip mats and grab bars in the bathtub.
- Remove electrical cords that extend across the floor.
- Remove throw rugs.
- Keep a flashlight near your bed for emergencies.
- Avoid climbing onto step stool and ladders.
- Avoid rushing to the phone to answer calls. Have a cordless phone.

Suggested Menu

Breakfast
Have 1 serving Fluffy Orange Pancakes leftover from Day 45. Serve with 1 cup fat-free milk and 1 cup red grapes.

Lunch
Have 1 serving Lime Peanut Salad leftover from Day 47. Serve with 1 cup low fat vanilla yogurt.

Snack
Have 1 sliced peach and 2 sliced apricots and top with 1 serving Sweet Cream Spread leftover from Day 46.

Dinner
Have 1 serving Lemon Lime Salmon with Asparagus. (Make whole recipe; save ½ for Day 49.) For dessert, have ½ cup of ice cream topped with 4 tbsp whipped cream and 1 tbsp chopped walnuts.

Daily Calorie total: 1551
Fat, 56 g % of daily cal: 32%
Saturated Fat, 17 g % of daily cal: 10%
Carbohydrate, 202 g % of daily cal: 52%
Protein, 77 g % of daily cal: 20%
Fiber, 21 g
Cholesterol, 241 mg
Calcium, 1250 mg
Sodium, 1410 mg

Breakfast

What I ate _____

What I was doing while I ate

Hunger level: **1** **2** **3** **4** **5**
Full / Starving

Lunch

What I ate _____

What I was doing while I ate

Hunger level: **1** **2** **3** **4** **5**
Full / Starving

Dinner

What I ate _____

What I was doing while I ate

Hunger level: **1** **2** **3** **4** **5**
Full / Starving

Snack (if desired)

What I ate _____

What I was doing while I ate

Hunger level: **1** **2** **3** **4** **5**
Full / Starving

Activity Map

Skin Fitness and Your Diet

A study in the *Journal of the American College of Nutrition* found "that skin wrinkling in a sun-exposed site in older people of various ethnic backgrounds may be influenced by the types of foods consumed." They found certain foods were associated with less skin damage, such as eggs, yogurt, legumes (especially broad and lima beans), vegetables (especially green leafy/spinach, eggplant, asparagus, celery, onions/leeks, garlic), nuts, olives, cherries, melon, dried fruits/prunes, apples/pears, multigrain bread, jam, tea, and water.

Your Bodyweight:_____

From Z and Tracy: Did you look in the mirror today? No! Go ahead we'll wait... Well, don't you feel and look better? All right now, we didn't say perfect. You might want to think about new clothes very soon since those inches are coming off. Have a great day today.

Aerobic Training Exercises

Always start your aerobic activity slowly and gradually progress to your target intensity. Choose one the following aerobic activities and do it for 30 to 45 minutes at an OMNI RPE of 5 to 7.

- Walking (outdoor or indoor)
- Biking (outdoor or indoor)
- Pool walking or exercises or swimming
- Dancing (such as salsa)
- Sports (such as tennis)

Stretching Exercises

Perform all of the following stretching exercises for 1 to 3 sets of 15 to 30 seconds.

- Wrist stretch
- Neck stretches
- Hands behind back stretch
- Hands behind head stretch
- Yawn stretch
- Look over the shoulder stretch
- Calf stretch
- Hip flexor stretch
- Hamstring stretch
- Quadriceps stretch
- Inner hip stretch
- Outer hip stretch

Relaxation

Finish your exercise program by lying down and doing the slow relaxation breathing technique for 1 to 5 minutes. You can also perform Tai Chi or Qi Gong as your cool down.

Did You Know That...

Humans have historically squatted during a bowel movement. The sitting posture assumed in Western cultures requires more effort for a bowel movement, which may lead to a serious strain to the heart and brain blood vessels, so stay regular and avoid holding your breath.

Nutrition Diary

Challenge Yourself – Try Qi Gong

Qi Gong is an ancient Chinese martial art that helps to improve relaxation, mental concentration, flexibility, and strength. Qi Gong is traditional Chinese movement therapy. Qi is the Chinese word for "life energy" and Gong means "work." Contact a local martial arts studio and take a few classes to see if this is a method you want to explore further.

Breakfast

What I ate _____

_____

What I was doing while I ate

_____

Hunger level: **1** **2** **3** **4** **5**
  Full   Starving

Lunch

What I ate _____

_____

What I was doing while I ate

_____

Hunger level: **1** **2** **3** **4** **5**
  Full   Starving

Dinner

What I ate _____

_____

What I was doing while I ate

_____

Hunger level: **1** **2** **3** **4** **5**
  Full   Starving

Snack (if desired)

What I ate _____

_____

What I was doing while I ate

_____

Hunger level: **1** **2** **3** **4** **5**
  Full   Starving

Suggested Menu

Breakfast
Have 1 Very Berry Smoothie.

Lunch
Have 1 serving Lemon Lime Salmon with Asparagus leftover from Day 48. Serve with ½ cup cooked whole wheat pasta topped with ¼ cup spaghetti sauce. Serve with a side of 10 grape tomatoes.

Snack
Have the last serving of Fluffy Orange Pancakes leftover from Day 46. Serve with 1 cup cubed cantaloupe.

Dinner
Have 1 serving Scallops with Kumquat Chutney. (Make whole recipe; save ½ for Day 50.) For dessert, have 1 low fat ice cream sandwich.

Daily Calorie total: 1576
Fat, 44 g % of daily cal: 25%
Saturated Fat, 9 g % of daily cal: 5%
Carbohydrate, 211 g % of daily cal: 54%
Protein, 94 g % of daily cal: 24%
Fiber, 32 g
Cholesterol, 233 mg
Calcium, 1269 mg
Sodium, 1428 mg

Activity Map

Seasonal Fitness

The following are some general suggestions to encourage you to think about a variety of ways you can be active during the year.

Winter
- Go skiing.
- Go sled riding.
- Go ice skating.

Spring
- Play basketball.
- Go bike riding.
- Shoot a round of golf.

Summer
- Play softball.
- Play volleyball.
- Go swimming.

Autumn
- Play tennis.
- Play touch football.

From Z and Tracy: Last week and then we reassess your goals. We're fairly confident that you'll be happy with the results. Talk to you soon.

Aerobic Training Exercises

Always start your aerobic activity slowly and gradually progress to your target intensity. Choose one the following aerobic activities and do it for 30 to 45 minutes at an OMNI RPE of 5 to 7.

- Walking (outdoor or indoor)
- Biking (outdoor or indoor)
- Pool walking or exercises or swimming
- Dancing (such as salsa)
- Sports (such as tennis)

Stretching Exercises

Perform all of the following stretching exercises for 1 to 3 sets of 15 to 30 seconds.

- Wrist stretch
- Neck stretches
- Hands behind back stretch
- Hands behind head stretch
- Yawn stretch
- Look over the shoulder stretch
- Calf stretch
- Hip flexor stretch
- Hamstring stretch
- Quadriceps stretch
- Inner hip stretch
- Outer hip stretch

Relaxation

Finish your exercise program by lying down and doing the slow relaxation breathing technique for 1 to 5 minutes. You can also perform Tai Chi or Qi Gong as your cool down.

Nutrition Diary

Eating Out and About with Ease

Here are a few ideas to control your portions and calories when you're eating out:

• Have a general plan of what you want to order before you get to the restaurant. For example, if you want a piece of steak, plan ahead for low-fat sides such as steamed vegetables and a baseball-size portion of starch such as rice, a baked potato or bread, not all three.

• If you're worried about oversized portions, order from the a la carte menu. It's easy to put together a nice meal with a chicken kabob appetizer, a side salad, a steamed vegetable of the day, and a baked potato.

Suggested Menu

Breakfast
Have 1 serving Fruit and Cheese Foldover. Serve with 1 cup fat-free milk.

Lunch
Have 1 serving Scallops with Kumquat Chutney leftover from Day 49.

Snack
Toast ½ of a 6" whole wheat pita bread, cut into triangles, dip into one serving Peanutty Ricotta Spread leftover from Day 25. (Save the other ½ of the pita bread for Day 51.)

Dinner
Have 1 serving Asian Mixed Green Salad with Persimmons. (Make whole recipe; save ½ for Day 51.) For dessert, have 1 Frozen Milk Pop.

Daily Calorie total: 1634
Fat, 39 g % of daily cal: 21%
Saturated Fat, 12 g % of daily cal: 7%
Carbohydrate, 239 g % of daily cal: 59 %
Protein, 96 g % of daily cal: 24%
Fiber, 27 g
Cholesterol, 166 mg
Calcium, 1194 mg
Sodium, 2320 mg

Breakfast

What I ate _____

_____

What I was doing while I ate

_____

Hunger level: **1**   **2**   **3**   **4**   **5**
           Full   Starving

Lunch

What I ate _____

_____

What I was doing while I ate

_____

Hunger level: **1**   **2**   **3**   **4**   **5**
           Full   Starving

Dinner

What I ate _____

_____

What I was doing while I ate

_____

Hunger level: **1**   **2**   **3**   **4**   **5**
           Full   Starving

Snack (if desired)

What I ate _____

_____

What I was doing while I ate

_____

Hunger level: **1**   **2**   **3**   **4**   **5**
           Full   Starving

the **Anti-Aging Fitness**
PRESCRIPTION

Activity Map

Gym Fitness– Choosing a Gym

Look for the following key factors when choosing a gym:

• Is the location near your home or work?

• What is the training of the professional fitness staff?

• Does the gym have a good reputation for quality service?

• Do the hours of operation fit your schedule?

• Is the cost reasonable?

• Do they have equipment and features that appeal to you?

• Do they offer classes (such as Yoga, Tai Chi, Pilates)?

• Do you like the atmosphere?

We suggest you ask for a free or paid guest pass and first try the gym for one or more visits before investing into any type of membership.

266

Warm Up Exercises

Perform all of the following warm up exercises for 1 set of 10 reps for each exercise.

• March in place
• Shake, rattle and roll
• Trunk rotations
• Lower back cat / camel

• Heel sits with arms in front
• Heel sits with arms to side
• Hip windshield wiper

Strength Training Exercises

Perform all of the following muscle building and toning exercises for 2 to 3 sets of 8 to 15 reps.

• Wall ball squats
• Heel raises
• Partial step-ups
• Elastic pull to chest
• Elastic outward rotation
• Dumbbell overhead press

• Modified pushups
• Elastic triceps pushdown
• Dumbbell biceps curl
• Side bridging
• Exercise ball abdominal curls
• Pelvic floor contract, hold, release

Balance Exercises

Perform both balance exercises for 1 to 3 sets of 30 to 60 seconds.

• Very slow motion balancing and walking in place
• Dancer's balance

Stretching Exercises

Perform all of the following stretching exercises for 1 to 3 sets of 15 to 30 seconds.

• Wrist stretch
• Neck stretches
• Hands behind back stretch
• Hands behind head stretch
• Yawn stretch
• Look over the shoulder stretch

• Calf stretch
• Hip flexor stretch
• Hamstring stretch
• Quadriceps stretch
• Inner hip stretch
• Outer hip stretch

Relaxation

Finish your exercise program by lying down and doing the slow relaxation breathing technique for 1 to 5 minutes. You can also perform Tai Chi or Qi Gong as your cool down.

Nutrition Diary

Steer Clear

Be wary of anything on the menu labeled as follows. The dishes may sound glamorous, but their effects on your body are anything but!

Agemono: Fried – Steer Clear

Alfredo: Prepared with cream, butter and cheese – Steer Clear

Con queso: With cheese – Ask for no cheese or use an ounce or about the amount in a pair of dice.

Country-style: Most likely means fried, battered or smothered in gravy, Steer Clear

Escalloped: Thinly sliced and prepared with a creamy sauce – Steer Clear

Frito or Fritto: Fried – Steer Clear

Breakfast

What I ate _____

_____

What I was doing while I ate

_____

Hunger level: **1**   **2**   **3**   **4**   **5**
                  Full   Starving

Lunch

What I ate _____

_____

What I was doing while I ate

_____

Hunger level: **1**   **2**   **3**   **4**   **5**
                  Full   Starving

Dinner

What I ate _____

_____

What I was doing while I ate

_____

Hunger level: **1**   **2**   **3**   **4**   **5**
                  Full   Starving

Snack (if desired)

What I ate _____

_____

What I was doing while I ate

_____

Hunger level: **1**   **2**   **3**   **4**   **5**
                  Full   Starving

Suggested Menu

Breakfast
Have 1 serving Sweet Cottage Cheese Bowl. Serve with 1 cup fat-free milk.

Lunch
Have 1 serving Asian Mixed Green Salad leftover from Day 50.

Snack
Have ½ whole wheat pita bread leftover from Day 50. Toast it, cut into triangles and dip into 1 serving Peanuty Ricotta Spread leftover from Day 25.

Dinner
Have 1 serving Baked Acorn Squash. (Make whole recipe; save ½ for Day 52.) Have 1 Tasty Turkey Burger. (Make ½ of recipe, and save ½ for Day 52.) Top turkey burger with ½ tomato (save the other ½ for Day 52) and 2 tbsp ketchup and mustard if desired. For dessert, have 1 serving Pudding Parfait. (Make the whole box of pudding, assemble parfaits just before eating. Save leftover for Days 52, 53 and 54.)

Daily Calorie total: 1579
Fat, 26 g % of daily cal: 15%
Saturated Fat, 10 g % of daily cal: 6%
Carbohydrate, 233 g % of daily cal: 59%
Protein, 117 g % of daily cal: 30%
Fiber, 24 g
Cholesterol, 163 mg
Calcium, 1159 mg
Sodium, 3354 mg

theAnti-Aging Fitness
PRESCRIPTION

Activity Map

Gym Fitness – Starting Out

When you do finally select a gym, have a personal trainer guide you through the following simple gym program to get you started:

• Warm up slowly on a bike or treadmill.

• Do leg press machine.

• Do rowing machine.

• Do lat pulldown machine.

• Do chest press machine.

• Do cable triceps push-down machine.

• Do dumbbell biceps curl.

• Cool down slowly on a bike or treadmill and then stretch.

Do the above program 2 to 3 times a week. On separate days you can do an aerobic exercise on a bike or treadmill for 30 to 45 minutes.

Aerobic Training Exercises

Always start your aerobic activity slowly and gradually progress to your target intensity. Choose one the following aerobic activities and do it for 30 to 45 minutes at an OMNI RPE of 5 to 7.

• Walking (outdoor or indoor)
• Biking (outdoor or indoor)
• Pool walking or exercises or swimming
• Dancing (such as salsa)
• Sports (such as tennis)

Stretching Exercises

Perform all of the following stretching exercises for 1 to 3 sets of 15 to 30 seconds.

• Wrist stretch
• Neck stretches
• Hands behind back stretch
• Hands behind head stretch
• Yawn stretch
• Look over the shoulder stretch
• Calf stretch
• Hip flexor stretch
• Hamstring stretch
• Quadriceps stretch
• Inner hip stretch
• Outer hip stretch

Relaxation

Finish your exercise program by lying down and doing the slow relaxation breathing technique for 1 to 5 minutes. You can also perform Tai Chi or Qi Gong as your cool down.

Nutrition Diary

Enjoy Eating Out

Au Fines Herbes: Coated in chopped herbs, usually parsley, tarragon, chives or chervil – Enjoy!

Au gratin: Topped with cheese and buttered bread crumbs – If you can take off some of the topping, go ahead and enjoy half.

Au Jus: Pan juice or broth, often with no added fat – Enjoy!

Encrusted: Typically means coated with nuts or bread crumbs and often pan-fried – Ask the server to use less than half of the oil.

Reduction: Stock, wine or light sauce that has been concentrated – Enjoy!

Breakfast

What I ate _____

_____

What I was doing while I ate

_____

Hunger level: **1**   **2**   **3**   **4**   **5**
    Full   Starving

Lunch

What I ate _____

_____

What I was doing while I ate

_____

Hunger level: **1**   **2**   **3**   **4**   **5**
    Full   Starving

Dinner

What I ate _____

_____

What I was doing while I ate

_____

Hunger level: **1**   **2**   **3**   **4**   **5**
    Full   Starving

Snack (if desired)

What I ate _____

_____

What I was doing while I ate

_____

Hunger level: **1**   **2**   **3**   **4**   **5**
    Full   Starving

Suggested Menu

Breakfast
Have 6 graham cracker squares dipped into 1 serving Peanuty Ricotta Spread leftover from Day 50. Freeze remainder for up to a month. Serve with 1 pear and 1 cup fat-free milk.

Lunch
Have 1 serving Baked Acorn Squash and 1 Tasty Turkey Burger leftover from Day 51. Top turkey burger with ½ tomato leftover from Day 51 and 2 tbsp ketchup and mustard if desired.

Snack
Serve 1 Pria bar with ½ sliced mango, save ½ for Day 53.

Dinner
Have 1 serving Broccoli, Beef and Tomatoes. (Make whole recipe; save ½ for Day 53.) For dessert, have 1 serving Pudding Parfait leftover from Day 51.

Daily Calorie total: 1625
Fat, 41 g % of daily cal: 23%
Saturated Fat, 16 g % of daily cal: 9%
Carbohydrate, 230 g % of daily cal: 57%
Protein, 102 g % of daily cal: 25%
Fiber, 28 g
Cholesterol, 153 mg
Calcium, 1126 mg
Sodium, 2085 mg

269

the **Anti-Aging Fitness**
PRESCRIPTION

Activity Map

Outdoor Adventure Fitness

You've exercised in your home, pool and gym and now you're looking for some adventure. Try the following outdoor activities for variety:

- Canoeing
- Horseback riding
- Kayaking
- Mountain biking
- Rafting
- Rock climbing
- Sailing
- Scuba diving
- Skiing
- Surfing
- Windsurfing

Aerobic Training Exercises

Always start your aerobic activity slowly and gradually progress to your target intensity. Choose one the following aerobic activities and do it for 30 to 45 minutes at an OMNI RPE of 5 to 7.

- Walking (outdoor or indoor)
- Biking (outdoor or indoor)
- Pool walking or exercises or swimming
- Dancing (such as salsa)
- Sports (such as tennis)

Stretching Exercises

Perform all of the following stretching exercises for 1 to 3 sets of 15 to 30 seconds.

- Wrist stretch
- Neck stretches
- Hands behind back stretch
- Hands behind head stretch
- Yawn stretch
- Look over the shoulder stretch
- Calf stretch
- Hip flexor stretch
- Hamstring stretch
- Quadriceps stretch
- Inner hip stretch
- Outer hip stretch

Relaxation

Finish your exercise program by lying down and doing the slow relaxation breathing technique for 1 to 5 minutes. You can also perform Tai Chi or Qi Gong as your cool down.

Nutrition Diary

Holiday Fitness

Stay active during the holidays to prevent weight gain.

New Years: Start the new year off by walking with a friend.

Memorial Day: Take the family to the pool.

4th Of July: Play a softball game as a part of the picnic.

Labor Day: Take the family and friends for a camping trip.

Thanksgiving: Before the big dinner play a game of touch football or go for a walk. After the dinner and several football games, go for a walk to help improve digestion and work off some calories.

Breakfast

What I ate _____

_____

What I was doing while I ate

_____

Hunger level: **1**   **2**   **3**   **4**   **5**
                Full   Starving

Lunch

What I ate _____

_____

What I was doing while I ate

_____

Hunger level: **1**   **2**   **3**   **4**   **5**
                Full   Starving

Dinner

What I ate _____

_____

What I was doing while I ate

_____

Hunger level: **1**   **2**   **3**   **4**   **5**
                Full   Starving

Snack (if desired)

What I ate _____

_____

What I was doing while I ate

_____

Hunger level: **1**   **2**   **3**   **4**   **5**
                Full   Starving

Suggested Menu

Breakfast
Have 1 serving Tropical Cereal. Serve with 1 12 oz. nonfat latte and 1½ cups cubed watermelon.

Lunch
Have 1 serving Broccoli, Beef and Tomato leftover from Day 52. Serve with 1 cup raw baby carrots.

Snack
Slice an apple and dip into 1 serving of Spicy Pumpkin Dip leftover from Day 29.

Dinner
Have 1 serving Fast Falafel. For dessert, have 1 serving Pudding Parfait leftover from Day 51.

Daily Calorie total: 1639
Fat, 38 g % of daily cal: 21%
Saturated Fat, 8 g % of daily cal: 5%
Carbohydrate, 272 g % of daily cal: 66%
Protein, 73 g % of daily cal: 20%
Fiber, 42 g
Cholesterol, 41 mg
Calcium, 1630 mg
Sodium, 2252 mg

271

the**Anti-Aging Fitness**
PRESCRIPTION

Activity Map

Pool Fitness

Exercising in the water is a great way to add variety to your workouts. It can also be an excellent program if you have arthritis or recovering from back, hip or knee surgery.

Try the following simple program in chest or shoulder deep water:

• Warm up slowly by walking back and forth in the pool.

• Do partial knee bends.

• Do heel raises.

• Do single leg balancing.

• Do an alternate pushing and pulling motion with your arms.

• Do marching in place.

• Cool down slowly by walking back and forth and then stretch.

Caution: Never swim alone just in case you need help.

Warm Up Exercises

Perform all of the following warm up exercises for 1 set of 10 reps for each exercise.

• March in place
• Shake, rattle and roll
• Trunk rotations
• Lower back cat / camel

• Heel sits with arms in front
• Heel sits with arms to side
• Hip windshield wiper

Strength Training Exercises

Perform all of the following muscle building and toning exercises for 2 to 3 sets of 8 to 15 reps at an OMNI RPE of 5 to 7.

• Wall ball squats
• Heel raises
• Partial step-ups
• Elastic pull to chest
• Elastic outward rotation
• Dumbbell overhead press

• Modified pushups
• Elastic triceps pushdown
• Dumbbell biceps curl
• Side bridging
• Exercise ball abdominal curls
• Pelvic floor contract, hold, release

Balance Exercises

Perform both balance exercises for 1 to 3 sets of 30 to 60 seconds.

• Very slow motion balancing and walking in place

• Dancer's balance

Stretching Exercises

Perform all of the following stretching exercises for 1 to 3 sets of 15 to 30 seconds.

• Wrist stretch
• Neck stretches
• Hands behind back stretch
• Hands behind head stretch
• Yawn stretch
• Look over the shoulder stretch

• Calf stretch
• Hip flexor stretch
• Hamstring stretch
• Quadriceps stretch
• Inner hip stretch
• Outer hip stretch

Relaxation

Finish your exercise program by lying down and doing the slow relaxation breathing technique for 1 to 5 minutes. You can also perform Tai Chi or Qi Gong as your cool down.

Nutrition Diary

Holiday Eating Tips

Have a plan for handling holiday party eating. Choose what splurges will give you the most satisfaction, whether it's the buttery cookie, fudge or a slice of frosted cake. Here are some tips for keeping your hands and your mouth busy:

• Keep a drink in your hand at all times. Choose sparkling water with a lemon or lime, diet soda or tea. It's a little harder to pick up food when you have to put your drink down.

• For ladies, carry a clutch purse and a drink, this way neither hand is free to nibble needlessly.

• Make a point to circulate around a party and speak to everyone. It may take your mind off eating more.

Suggested Menu

Breakfast
Have 1 serving Feta Broccoli Fritatta. (Make ½ of recipe.) Serve with 1 cup fat-free milk and 2 kiwi.

Lunch
Have 1 serving Spring Green Walnut Salad (make ½ of recipe).

Snack
Have 1 low fat vanilla yogurt, topped with 3 tbsp chopped walnuts.

Dinner
Have 1 serving Pasta Primavera. (Make whole recipe; save ½ for Day 55.) For dessert, have 1 serving Pudding Parfait leftover from Day 51.

Daily Calorie total: 1563
Fat, 60 g % of daily cal: 35%
Saturated Fat, 16 g % of daily cal: 9%
Carbohydrate, 193 g % of daily cal: 49%
Protein, 80 g % of daily cal: 20%
Fiber, 33 g
Cholesterol, 145 mg
Calcium, 1354 mg
Sodium, 2421 mg

Breakfast

What I ate _____

_____

What I was doing while I ate

_____

Hunger level: **1** **2** **3** **4** **5**
     Full   Starving

Lunch

What I ate _____

_____

What I was doing while I ate

_____

Hunger level: **1** **2** **3** **4** **5**
     Full   Starving

Dinner

What I ate _____

_____

What I was doing while I ate

_____

Hunger level: **1** **2** **3** **4** **5**
     Full   Starving

Snack (if desired)

What I ate _____

_____

What I was doing while I ate

_____

Hunger level: **1** **2** **3** **4** **5**
     Full   Starving

273

the Anti-Aging Fitness
PRESCRIPTION

Activity Map

Travel Fitness?

Sitting in prolonged positions may lead to swelling in the feet, back stiffness and increases the risk for deep vein thrombosis (a blood clot in one or more of the deep veins of the legs arms, pelvis, neck, axilla, or chest). This problem, commonly associated with long haul travel, has been called "coach class" or "traveler's thrombosis." Move your legs when you are in confined places for prolonged periods such as when traveling in an airplane, car, bus, and train.

Ideally try to stand and walk around every 20 to 50 minutes after sitting.

Aerobic Training Exercises

Always start your aerobic activity slowly and gradually progress to your target intensity. Choose one the following aerobic activities and do it for 30 to 45 minutes at an OMNI RPE of 5 to 7.

- Walking (outdoor or indoor)
- Biking (outdoor or indoor)
- Pool walking or exercises or swimming
- Dancing (such as salsa)
- Sports (such as tennis)

Stretching Exercises

Perform all of the following stretching exercises for 1 to 3 sets of 15 to 30 seconds.

- Wrist stretch
- Neck stretches
- Hands behind back stretch
- Hands behind head stretch
- Yawn stretch
- Look over the shoulder stretch
- Calf stretch
- Hip flexor stretch
- Hamstring stretch
- Quadriceps stretch
- Inner hip stretch
- Outer hip stretch

Relaxation

Finish your exercise program by lying down and doing the slow relaxation breathing technique for 1 to 5 minutes. You can also perform Tai Chi or Qi Gong as your cool down.

Anti-Aging Hint:

Good posture is dynamic and means you vary it periodically to avoid excess physical stress to one area. So stay loose and relaxed.

274

Nutrition Diary

Holiday Time Management

The holidays can be stressful. Even the most dedicated of us may find it tough to stick to our regular plan. Your new lifestyle should take priority, and your efforts to get enough sleep, eat healthy and exercise will help you handle the stress of travel and family interaction. Some tips:

• Stick to regular mealtimes as much as possible. Skipping meals to "bank" calories for a splurge can backfire.

• Never sacrifice sleep for gift wrapping, cooking or party planning. Plan a few days in advance and make and freeze foods if possible, wrap a few gifts each night and keep the decorations simple.

• If you're crunched for time, opt for a shorter workout. A little workout is better than none at all!

Breakfast

What I ate _____

_____

What I was doing while I ate

_____

Hunger level: **1**   **2**   **3**   **4**   **5**
                Full   Starving

Lunch

What I ate _____

_____

What I was doing while I ate

_____

Hunger level: **1**   **2**   **3**   **4**   **5**
                Full   Starving

Dinner

What I ate _____

_____

What I was doing while I ate

_____

Hunger level: **1**   **2**   **3**   **4**   **5**
                Full   Starving

Snack (if desired)

What I ate _____

_____

What I was doing while I ate

_____

Hunger level: **1**   **2**   **3**   **4**   **5**
                Full   Starving

Suggested Menu
Breakfast
Serve 1 slice of pumpernickel toast topped with 2 tbsp crumbled feta cheese and 5 halved grape tomatoes. Have 1 cup low fat plain yogurt mixed with 1 fresh pomegranate.
Lunch
Have 1 serving Chili leftover from Day 27.
Snack
Have 1 Very Berry Smoothie.
Dinner
Have 1 serving Pasta Primavera leftover from Day 54. For dessert, have 1 low fat ice cream sandwich.

Daily Calorie total: 1531
Fat, 56 g % of daily cal: 33%
Saturated Fat, 17 g % of daily cal: 10%
Carbohydrate, 188 g % of daily cal: 49%
Protein, 87 g % of daily cal: 23%
Fiber, 33 g
Cholesterol, 275 mg
Calcium, 1773 mg
Sodium, 2244 mg

275

the **Anti-Aging Fitness**
PRESCRIPTION

Activity Map

Proper Care Leads To A Healthy Smile

Avoid smoking and keep alcohol consumption at moderate levels to prevent periodontal disease and oral cancer. Keeping your mouth healthy can also prevent pain and difficulty with chewing foods and not limit your foods choices. A study in the *Journal of the American Dietetic Association* showed that individuals with oral health problems had lower dietary intakes of vitamin A, C and B 6. So, brush, floss, get regular dental checkups and eat fresh wholesome foods to keep your teeth and gums healthy.

Your Bodyweight:_____

From Z and Tracy: 8 weeks!! We're very proud of you for staying with us. We hope that when you check your goals that you've made big strides in accomplishing them.

Warm Up Exercises

Perform all of the following warm up exercises for 1 set of 10 reps for each exercise.
- March in place
- Shake, rattle and roll
- Trunk rotations
- Lower back cat / camel
- Heel sits with arms in front
- Heel sits with arms to side
- Hip windshield wiper

Strength Training Exercises

Perform all of the following muscle building and toning exercises for 2 to 3 sets of 8 to 15 reps at an OMNI RPE of 5 to 7.
- Wall ball squats
- Heel raises
- Partial step-ups
- Elastic pull to chest
- Elastic outward rotation
- Dumbbell overhead press
- Modified pushups
- Elastic triceps pushdown
- Dumbbell biceps curl
- Side bridging
- Exercise ball abdominal curls
- Pelvic floor contract, hold, release

Balance Exercises

Perform both balance exercises for 1 to 3 sets of 30 to 60 seconds.
- Very slow motion balancing and walking in place
- Dancer's balance

Stretching Exercises

Perform all of the following stretching exercises for 1 to 3 sets of 15 to 30 seconds.
- Wrist stretch
- Neck stretches
- Hands behind back stretch
- Hands behind head stretch
- Yawn stretch
- Look over the shoulder stretch
- Calf stretch
- Hip flexor stretch
- Hamstring stretch
- Quadriceps stretch
- Inner hip stretch
- Outer hip stretch

Relaxation

Finish your exercise program by lying down and doing the slow relaxation breathing technique for 1 to 5 minutes. You can also perform Tai Chi or Qi Gong as your cool down.

276

Nutrition Diary

Revisiting Your Goals

Back on Day 7, you mapped out some goals. How did you do? As you end your 8-week plan, think about the new steps you'll take to continue your healthy habits. Are there exercises you'd like to try or lessons you'd like to take? If you've been wanting to take ballroom dance lessons or join a master's swim club, go ahead and write it down. Research your options to make it happen. You can make the most of your life, start with setting a plan today to do something you've always wanted to do.

I plan to follow these steps to better health ...

1. _____

2. _____

3. _____

Breakfast

What I ate _____

_____

What I was doing while I ate

_____

Hunger level: **1**   **2**   **3**   **4**   **5**
      Full   Starving

Lunch

What I ate _____

_____

What I was doing while I ate

_____

Hunger level: **1**   **2**   **3**   **4**   **5**
      Full   Starving

Dinner

What I ate _____

_____

What I was doing while I ate

_____

Hunger level: **1**   **2**   **3**   **4**   **5**
      Full   Starving

Snack (if desired)

What I ate _____

_____

What I was doing while I ate

_____

Hunger level: **1**   **2**   **3**   **4**   **5**
      Full   Starving

Suggested Menu

Breakfast

Have 1 serving Festival of Fruit Salad. Serve with 1 cup fat-free milk, 1 slice whole wheat toast topped with 1 slice soy cheese, bake in the oven at 250 degrees.

Lunch

Make a salad with 2 cups baby spinach leaves, 1 cup cubed honeydew, 1 ounce shredded Gouda cheese and 3 tbsp pecans. Top with 2 tbsp raspberry vinaigrette salad dressing. Serve with 10 small wheat crackers.

Snack

Have ½ cup heated vegetarian baked beans, top with 2 tbsp fat-free sour cream and scoop with 9 baked tortilla chips.

Dinner

Have 1 serving Pizza with Roasted Vegetables leftover from Day 34. Serve with ½ grapefruit. For dessert, have 1 regular fudgesicle.

Daily Calorie total: 1622
Fat, 55 g % of daily cal: 31%
Saturated Fat, 13 g % of daily cal: 7%
Carbohydrate, 245 g % of daily cal: 60%
Protein, 58 g % of daily cal: 14%
Fiber, 37 g
Cholesterol, 52 mg
Calcium, 1187 mg
Sodium, 1979 mg

Final Words from Z and Tracy

Congratulations in finishing your Eight-Week Anti-Aging Fitness Prescription. We hope you feel healthier so you can take on your life's challenges and pursue other personal goals. At this point, please reassess your goals. How well did you do? We hope excellent!

Now, go and take an "after" picture of yourself and paste it next to your "before" picture. We hope you're happy with the results. Remember though, it's not about how you look that's most important but rather how you feel.

For your future exercises, we want you to focus on having fun and just try to have a weekly balance of aerobic, strength, flexibility, and balance exercises. Of course, don't forget to challenge yourself with other activities such as dance, yoga, Tai Chi, or tennis. Expand your eating options with the Mix 'n Match Anti-Aging Meal Plan and this will help you keep on track with the three calcium-rich foods, at least three meals and the three various colored fruits and vegetables every day. We've included a generic Activity Map and Nutrition Diary page for you, which you can photocopy as many times as you need, so that you can continue to keep track of your progress. Once again, we thank you for taking this Eight-week journey with us.

Index of Exercises

Index of Recipes

Activity Map

Aerobic Training Exercises

Activity:

Time:

Intensity:

Strength Training Exercises

Exercises:

Sets:

Reps:

Intensity:

Stretching Exercises

Exercises:

Sets:

Time:

Balance Exercises

Exercises:

Sets:

Time:

Date:

Nutrition Diary

Breakfast

What I ate _____

_____

What I was doing while I ate

_____

Hunger level: **1**   **2**   **3**   **4**   **5**
           Full   Starving

Lunch

What I ate _____

_____

What I was doing while I ate

_____

Hunger level: **1**   **2**   **3**   **4**   **5**
           Full   Starving

Dinner

What I ate _____

_____

What I was doing while I ate

_____

Hunger level: **1**   **2**   **3**   **4**   **5**
           Full   Starving

Three Different-Colored Vegetables:

1.

2.

3.

Three Different-Colored Fruits:

1.

2.

3.

Three Calcium-Rich Foods:

1.

2.

3.

Snack (if desired)

What I ate _____

_____

What I was doing while I ate

_____

Hunger level: **1**   **2**   **3**   **4**   **5**
           Full   Starving

Four Wholesome Carbs:

1.

2.

3.

4.

Four of the Finest Fats:

1.

2.

3.

4.

Six Lean, Mean Proteins

1.

2.

3.

4.

5.

6.

Daily Calorie Total:

theAnti-Aging Fitness
PRESCRIPTION

Resources and Further Readings

Associations

Contact the following organizations to obtain more information about specific health related topic.

American Academy of Dermatology
www.aad.org

American Academy of Ophthalmology
www.aao.org

American Association of Colleges of Osteopathic Medicine
www.aacom.org

American Association of Retired Persons
www.aarp.org

American Aging Association
www.americanaging.org

American Cancer Society
www.cancer.org

American College of Rheumatology
www.rheumatology.org

American College of Sports Medicine
www.acsm.org

American Diabetes Association
www.diabetes.org

American Dietetic Association
www.eatright.org

American Federation for Aging Research
www.infoaging.org

American Heart Association
www.americanheart.org

American Institute of Stress
www.stress.org

American Occupational Therapy Association
www.aota.org

American Physical Therapy Association
www.apta.org

American Society on Aging
www.asaging.org

American Stroke Association
www.strokeassociation.org

Arthritis Foundation
www.arthritis.org

Mind Body Medical Institute
www.mbmi.org

National Institute on Aging
www.nia.nih.org

National Osteoporosis Foundation
www.nof.org

National Sleep Foundation
www.sleepfoundation.org

National Strength and Conditioning Association
www.nsca-lift.org

Medical Research

Use the following to do some of your own research into a particular topic to supplement the information provided by your healthcare provider.

American Medical Association
www.ama-assn.org

Center for Disease Control and Prevention
www.cdc.gov

Cochrane Collaboration
www.cochrane.org

eMedicine
www.emedicine.com

Food and Drug Administration
www.fda.gov

Merck Manual
www.merck.com

National Academy of Sciences — Institute of Medicine
www.iom.edu

National Blueprint
www.agingblueprint.org

National Institutes of Health (NIH)
www.nih.gov

United States National Library of Medicine
www.nlm.nih.gov

WebMD.com
www.webmd.com

World Health Organization
www.who.int

Product Resources

Use the following resources to find products and equipment.

Cramer (sports medicine products)
www.cramersportsmed.com

Flaghouse
(recreation and rehabilitation products)
www.flaghouse.com

Hydro-Fit
(aquatic exercise products)
www.hydrofit.com

Hydro-Tone
(aquatic exercise products)
www.hydrotone.com

Mueller Sports Medicine
(sports medicine products)
www.muellersportsmed.com

Perform Better
(sports medicine and fitness products)
www.performbetter.com

Speedo
(aquatic exercise products)
www.speedo.com

Sprint
(aquatic exercise products)
www.sprintaquatics.com

Thera-Band
(elastic resistance products)
www.thera-band.com

Further Readings

Try these books for more information about specific health topics.

Alexander FM. *The Use of The Self.* New York, NY: E. P. Dutton and Co., Inc., 1932.

Benson H, Klipper MZ. The Relaxation Response, New York, NY: Harper Torch, 1975.

Feldenkrais M. *Awareness Through Movement: Health Exercises for Personal Growth.* New York, NY: Harper & Row, 1972.

Holick MF, Jenkins M. *The UV Advantage.* New York, NY: ibooks, inc, 2004.

Jacobson E. *You Must Relax.* New York, NY: McGraw-Hill Book Company, Inc., 1962.

Jacobson E. *Progressive Relaxation, 4th ed.* Chicago, IL: University of Chicago Press, 1962.

Jones CJ, Rose DJ, eds. *Physical Activity Instruction of Older Adults.* Champaign, IL: Human Kinetics, 2005.

Kit WK. *The Complete Book of Tai Chi Chuan: A Comprehensive Guide To The Principles and Practice.* North Clarendon, VT: Tuttle Publishing, 2002.

Lasater J. *Relax and Renew.* Berkeley, CA: Rodmell Press, 1995.

Liu H, Perry P. *The Healing Art of Qi Gong.* New York, NY: Warner Books, 1997.

Schatz MP. *Back Care Basics: A Doctor's Gentle Yoga Program for Back and Neck Relief.* Berkeley, CA: Rodmell Press, 1992.

Selye H. *Stress in Health and Disease.* Boston, MA: Butterworths, 1976.

References

Chapter 1

AGING

The Centers for Disease Control and Prevention, http://www.cdc.gov, accessed October 2005.

The Department of Health and Human Services, Administration on Aging, http://www.aoa.dhhs.gov/press/pr/2003/05_m ay/ 05_29_03_pf.asp. October 2005.

The U.S. National Agricultural Library, http://www.nal.usda.gov/ fnic/Fpyr/pyramid.html, accessed October 2005.

SLEEP

American Sleep Apnea Association. http://www.sleepapnea.org/info/ index.html. accessed October 2005.

Ambrogio N, Cuttiford J, Lineker S, et al. A comparison of three types of neck support in fibromyalgia patients. *Arthritis Care and Research.* 1998;11(5):405-410.

Akita Y, Kawakatsu K, Hattori C, et al. Posture of patients with sleep apnea during sleep. *Acta otolaryngologica. Supplementum.* 2003;(550):41-45.

Ayas NT, White DP, Manson JE, et al. A prospective study of sleep duration and coronary heart disease in women. *Archives of Internal Medicine.* 2003;163(2):205-209.

Ayas NT, White DP, Al-Delaimy WK, et al. A prospective study of self-reported sleep duration and incident diabetes in women. *Diabetes Care.* 2003;26(2):380-384.

Connor J, Norton R, Ameratunga S, et al. Driver sleepiness and risk of serious injury to car occupants: Population based case control study. *British Medical Journal.* 2002;324(7346): 1125.

Dement WC. Some Must Watch While *Some Must Sleep: Exploring the World of Sleep.* New York, NY: W.W. Norton & Company, 1976.

Garfin SR, Pye SA. Bed design and its effect on chronic low back pain—a limited controlled trial. *Pain.* 1981;10(1):87-91.

Jacobson BH, Gemmell HA, Hayes BM, et al. Effectiveness of a selected bedding system on quality of sleep, low back pain, shoulder pain and spine stiffness. *Journal of Manipulative and Physiological Therapeutics.* 2002; 25(1):88-92.

Kelman BB. The sleep needs of adolescents. *Journal of School Nursing.* 1999;15(3):14-19.

Kovacs FM, Abraira V, Pena A, et al. Effect of firmness of mattress on chronic non-specific low-back pain: randomised, double-blind, controlled, multicentre trial. *Lancet.* 2003;362(9396): 1599-1604.

Kryger MH, Roth T, Dement WC. *Principles and Practice of Sleep Medicine,* 3rd ed. Philadelphia, PA: W.B. Saunders Company, 2000.

Lange T, Perras B, Fehm HL, et al. Sleep enhances the human antibody response to hepatitis A vaccination. *Psychosomatic Medicine.* 2003;65(5):831-835.

Lavin RA, Pappagallo M, Kuhlemeier KV. Cervical pain: A comparison of three pillows. *Archives of Physical Medicine and Rehabilitation.* 1997;78(2): 193-198.

Li F, Fisher KJ, Harmer P, et al. Tai chi and self-rated quality of sleep and daytime sleepiness in older adults: a randomized controlled trial. *Journal of the American Geriatrics Society.* 2004;52 (6):892-900.

Miyawaki S, Lavigne GJ, Pierre M, et al. Association between sleep bruxism, swallowing-related laryngeal movement, and sleep positions. *Sleep.* 2003;26(4): 461-465.

Persson L, Moritz U. Neck support pillows: A comparative study. *Journal of Manipulative and Physiological Therapeutics.* 1998;21 (4):237-240.

Spiegel K, Leproult R, Van Cauter E. Impact of sleep debt on metabolic and endocrine function. *Lancet* 1999;354 (9188): 1435-1439.

Van Dongen HPA, Maislin G, Mullington JM, et al. The cumulative cost of additional wakefulness: Dose-response effects on neurobehavioral functions and sleep physiology from chronic sleep restriction and total sleep deprivation. *Journal of Sleep and Sleep Disorders Research.* 2003;26(2): 117-126.

Walters PH. Sleep, the athlete, and performance. *Strength and Conditioning Journal.* 2002;24(2):17-24.

STRESS

Bennett MP, Zeller JM, Rosenberg L, et al. The effect of mirthful laughter on stress and natural killer cell activity. *Alternative Therapies in Health and Medicine.* 2003;9(2):38-45.

Bjorntorp P. Visceral fat accumulation: The missing link between psychosocial factors and cardiovascular disease? *Journal of Internal Medicine.* 1991;230(3): 195-201.

Bjorntorp P. Body fat distribution, insulin resistance, and metabolic diseases. *Nutrition.* 1997;13(9): 795-803.

Bjorntorp P, Rosmond R. Obesity and cortisol. *Nutrition.* 2000;16 (10):924-936.

Epel ES, Blackburn EH, Lin J, Dhabhar FS, et al. Accelerated telomere shortening in response to life stress. *Proceedings of the National Academy of Sciences of the United States of America.* 2004:101(49):17312- 17315.

Epel EE, Moyer AE, Martin CD, et al. Stress-induced cortisol, mood, and fat distribution in men. *Obesity Research.* 1999;7 (1):9-15.

Fox KR. The influence of physical activity on mental well-being. *Public Health Nutrition.* 1999;2 (3A):411-418.

Glaser R, Kiecolt-Glaser JK, Marucha PT, et al. Stress-related changes in proinflammatory cytokine production in wounds. *Archives of General Psychiatry.* 1999;56(5):450-456.

Hollmann W, Struder HK. Brain function, mind, nutrition, and physical exercise. *Nutrition.* 2000;16(7-8):516-519.

Irwin MR, Pike JL, Cole JC, et al. Effects of a behavioral intervention, tai chi chih, on varicella-zoster virus specific immunity and health functioning in older adults. *Psychosomatic Medicine.* 2003;65(5):824-830.

Jacks DE, Sowash J, Anning J, et al. Effect of exercise at three exercise intensities on salivary cortisol. *Journal of Strength and Conditioning Research.* 2002;16 (2):286-289.

Kiecolt-Glaser JK, Marucha PT, Malarkey WB, et al. Slowing of wound healing by psychological stress. *Lancet.* 1995;346 (8984):1194-1196.

Lombard CB. What is the role of food in preventing depression and improving mood, performance and cognitive function? *Medical Journal of Australia.* 2000;173(Suppl):S104-S105.

Oda S, Matsumoto T, Nakagawa K, et al. Relaxation effects in humans of underwater exercise of moderate intensity. *European Journal of Applied Physiology and Occupation Physiology.* 1999;80 (4):253-259.

Pawlow LA, O'Niel PM, Malcolm RJ. Night eating syndrome: effects of brief relaxation training on stress, mood, hunger and eating pattern. *International Journal Of Obesity And Related Metabolic Disorders.* 2003;27(8): 970-978.

Peeke P, Chrousos GP. Hypercortisolism and obesity. *Annals of the New York Academy of Sciences.* 1995;771:665-676.

Robles TF, Kiecolt-Glaser JK. The physiology of marriage: pathways to health. *Physiology and Behavior.* 2003;79(3):409-416.

Rosmond R, Bouchard C, Bjorntorp P. Tsp509I polymorphism in exon 2 of the glucocorticoid receptor gene in relation to obesity and cortisol secretion: Cohort study. *British Medical Journal.* 2001;322 (7287):652-653.

Selye H. *The Stress of Life,* revised edition. New York, NY: McGraw-Hill, 1976.

Selye H. *Stress Without Distress.* Philadelphia, PA: Lippincott, 1974.

Scully D, Kremer J, Meade MM, et al. Physical exercise and physiological well being: A critical review. *British Journal of Sports Medicine.* 1998;32(2):111-120.

Thoren P, Floras JS, Hoffmann P, et al. Endorphins and exercise: Physiological mechanisms and clinical implications. *Medicine and Science in Sports and Exercise.* 1990;22(4):417-428.

Venes D, ed. *Taber's Cyclopedic Medical Dictionary,* 19th ed. Philadelphia, PA: F.A. Davis Company, 2001.

Verrier RL, Mittleman MA. The impact of emotions on the heart. *Progress in Brain Research.* 2000;122: 369-380.

INFLAMMATION

Kimura H, Kimura M, Westra WH, et al. Increased thyroidal fat and goitrous hypothyroidism induced by interferon-gamma. *International Journal of Experimental Pathology.* 2005;86(2):97-106.

Petersen AM, Pedersen BK. The anti-inflammatory effect of exercise. *Journal of Applied Physiology.* 2005;98(4):1154-1162.

Steptoe A, Wardle J, Marmot M. Positive affect and health-related neuroendocrine, cardiovascular, and inflammatory processes. *Proceedings of the National Academy of Sciences of the United States of America.* 102(18):6508-6512.

Williams MJ, Milne BJ, Hancox RJ, et al. C-reactive protein and cardiorespiratory fitness in young adults. *European Journal of Cardiovascular Prevention and Rehabilitation.* 2005;12(3):216-220.

Wright CE, Strike PC, Brydon L, Steptoe A. Acute inflammation and negative mood: Mediation by cytokine activation. *Brain Behavior and Immunity.* 2005 Jul;19(4):345-50.

Chapter 2

Altug Z, Hoffman JL, Martin JL. *Manual of Clinical Exercise Testing, Prescription and Rehabilitation.* Norwalk, CT: Appleton & Lange, 1993.

American College of Sports Medicine. *ACSM's Resource Manual for Guidelines for Exercise Testing and Prescription, 5th ed.* Philadelphia, PA: Lippincott Williams & Wilkins, 2006.

American College of Sports Medicine. *ACSM's Guidelines for Exercise Testing and Prescription, 7th ed.* Philadelphia, PA: Lippincott Williams & Wilkins, 2005.

Astrand PO, Rodahl K, Dahl HA, et al. *Textbook of Work Physiology: Physiological Bases of Exercise,* 4th ed. Champaign, IL: Human Kinetics, 2003.

Heyward VH. Advanced *Fitness Assessment & Exercise Prescription,* 4th ed. Champaign, IL: Human Kinetics, 2002.

McArdle WD, Katch FI, Katch VL. *Exercise Physiology: Energy, Nutrition and Human Performance,* 5th ed. Baltimore, MD: Williams & Wilkins, 2001.

National Institutes of Health, National Heart, Lung, and Blood Institute and the National Institute of Diabetes and Digestive and Kidney Diseases. *Clinical Guidelines on the Identification, Evaluation, and Treatment of Overweight and Obesity in Adults: The Evidence Report.* Bethesda, MD: National Heart, Lung, and Blood Institute, 1998. NIH publication; No. 98-4083.

United States Department of Health and Human Services. *Physical Activity and Health: A Report of the Surgeon General.* Atlanta, GA: United States Department of Health and Human Services, 1996.

Chapter 3

WARM-UPS

Bishop D. Warm up I: Potential mechanisms and the effects of passive warm up on exercise performance. *Sports Medicine.* 2003;33(6):439-454.

Bishop D. Warm up II: Performance changes following active warm up and how to structure the warm up. *Sports Medicine.* 2003;33(7):483-498.

STRETCHING

Feland JB, Myrer JW, Schulthies SS, et al. The effect of duration of stretching of the hamstring muscle group for increasing range of motion in people aged 65 years or older. *Physical Therapy.* 2001;81(5):1110-1117.

Kendall FP, McCreary EK, Provance PG, et al. *Muscles: Testing and Function with Posture and Pain,* 5th ed. Baltimore, MD: Williams & Wilkins, 2005.

Sahrmann SA. *Diagnosis and Treatment of Movement Impairment Syndromes.* St. Louis, MO: Mosby, 2002.

Simons DG, Travell JG, Simons LS. *Travell & Simons' Myofascial Pain and Dysfunction: The Trigger Point Manual (Upper Half of Body),* 2nd ed. Volume 1. Baltimore, MD: Williams & Wilkins, 1999.

Travell JG, Simons DG. *Myofascial Pain and Dysfunc-*

tion: The Trigger Point Manual (Volume 1: The Lower Extremities). Baltimore, MD: Williams & Wilkins, 1992.

Chapter 4

Asplund CD, Brown DL. The running shoe prescription: fit for performance. *Physician and Sportsmedicine.* 2005;33(1):17-24.

Auble TE, Schwartz L. Physiological effects of exercising with handweights. *Sports Medicine.* 1991;11(4):244-256.

Brawner CA, Keteyian SJ, Czaplicki TE. A method for guiding exercise intensity: The talk test. *Medicine and Science in Sports and Exercise.* 1995;29:S241.

Brill J, Perry AC, Parker L, et al. Dose-response effect of walking exercise on weight loss. How much is enough? *International Journal of Obesity and Related Metabolic Disorders.* 2002; 26(11):1484-1493.

Brourman S. *Walk Yourself Well.* New York, NY: Hyperion, 1998.

Bryant DS, Goss FL, Robertson RJ, et al. Physiological responses to maximal treadmill and hand-weighted exercise. *Research Quarterly for Exercise and Sport.* 1993;64(3):300-304.

Felson DT (conference chair), et al. Osteoarthritis: New insights. Part 1: The disease and its risk factors. *Annals of Internal Medicine.* 2000;133(8):635-646.

Frey C. Foot health and shoewear for women. *Clinical Orthopaedics and Related Research.* 2000; (372):32-44.

Martin DR. Athletic shoes: Finding a good match.

Physician and Sportsmedicine. 1997;25(9):145-146.

Martin DR. How to steer patients toward the right sport shoe. *Physician and Sportsmedicine.* 1997;25(9):138-144.

McGill S. *Low Back Disorders: Evidence-Based Prevention and Rehabilitation.* Champaign, IL: Human Kinetics, 2002.

Murphy MH, Hardman AE. Training effects of short and long bouts of brisk walking in sedentary women. *Medicine and Science in Sports and Exercise.* 1998;30(1):152-157.

Murphy MH, Nevill AM, Hardman AE. Different patterns of brisk walking are equally effective in decreasing postprandial lipaedia. *International Journal of Obesity and Related Metabolic Disorders.* 2000;24(10):1303-1309.

Nesbitt L. How to buy athletic shoes. *Physician and Sportsmedicine.* 1999;27(12): 133-134.

Persinger R, Foster C, Gibson M, et al. Consistency of the talk test for exercise prescription. *Medicine and Science in Sports and Exercise.* 2004;36(9):1632-1636.

Schmidt WD, Biwer CJ, Kalscheuer LK. Effects of long versus short bout exercise on fitness and weight loss in overweight females. *Journal of the American College of Nutrition.* 2001;20(5):494-501.

Chapter 5

American College of Sports Medicine. ACSM's position stand: Progression models in resistance training for healthy adults. *Medicine & Science in Sports & Exercise.* 2002;34(2): 364-380.

Baechle TR, Earle RW, eds. *Essentials of Strength*

Training and Conditioning, 2nd ed. Champaign, IL: Human Kinetics, 2000.

Fiatarone MA, O'Neill EF, Ryan ND, et al. Exercise training and nutritional supplementation for physical frailty in very elderly people. *New England Journal of Medicine.* 1994;330(25):1769-1775.

Fiatarone MA, Marks EC, Ryan ND, et al. High-intensity strength training in nonagenarians. Effects on skeletal muscle. *Journal of the American Medical Association.* 1990;263(22):3029-3034.

Kegel A. Progressive resistance exercises in the functional restoration of the perineal muscles. *American Journal of Obstetrics and Gynecology.* 1948;56:238-249.

Kraemer WJ. Strength training basics: Designing workouts to meet patient's goals. *Physician and Sportsmedicine.* 2003;31 (8):39-45.

McGill S. *Low Back Disorders: Evidence-Based Prevention and Rehabilitation.* Champaign, IL: Human Kinetics, 2002.

McLester JR, Bishop P, Guilliams ME. Comparison of 1 day and 3 days per week of equal-volume resistance training in experienced subjects. *Journal of Strength and Conditioning Research.* 2000;14(3):273-281.

Noble E. *Essential Exercises for the Childbearing Year,* 4th ed. Harwich, MA: New Life Images, 2003.

Rhea MR, Alvar BA, Ball SD, et al. Three sets of weight training superior to 1 set with equal intensity for eliciting strength. *Journal of Strength and Conditioning Research.* 2002;16(4):525-529.

Richardson C, Hodges P, Hides J. *Therapeutic Exercise for Lumbopelvic Stabilization,* 2nd ed. Philadelphia, PA: Churchill Livingstone, 2004.

Seguin R, Nelson ME. Benefits of strength training for older adults. *American Journal of Preventive Medicine.* 2003;25(3Sii): 141-149.

Singh NA, Clements KM, Fiatarone MA. A randomized controlled trial of progressive resistance training in depressed elders. *Journals of Gerontology. Series A, Biological Sciences and Medical Sciences.* 1997;52(1): M27-35.

Spirduso WW, Francis KL, MacRae PG. *Physical Dimensions of Aging,* 2nd ed. Champaign, IL: Human Kinetics, 2005.

Chapter 6

United States National Agricultural Library, http://www.nal.usda.gov/ttic/tektran/category V3/Bioavailability.html, accessed October 2005.

Al-Hasso. Coenzyme Q10: a review. *Hospital Pharmacy.* 2001;36(1):51-66.

Ambrosone CB, McCann SE, Freudenheim JL, et al. Breast cancer risk in premenopausal women is inversely associated with consumption of broccoli, a source of isothiocyanates, but is not modified by GST genotype. *Journal of Nutrition.* 2004;134(5):1134-1138.

Ankri S, Mirelman D. Antimicrobial properties of allicin from garlic. *Microbes and Infection.* 1999;1(2):125-129.

Benton D. Selenium intake, mood and other aspects of psychological functioning. *Nutritional Neuroscience.* 2002 ;5(6):363-74.

Bohlke K, Spiegelman D, Trichopoulou A, et al. Vitamins A, C and E and the risk of breast cancer: results from a case-control study in Greece. *British Journal of Cancer.* 1999;79(1): 23-29.

Bonnefoy M, Drai J, Kostka T. Antioxidants to slow aging, facts and perspectives. *Presse Medicale.* 2002; 27;31(25):1174-84.

Broekmans WM, Klopping-Ketelaars IA, Schuurman CR, et al. Fruits and vegetables increase plasma carotenoids and vitamins and decrease homocysteine in humans. *Journal of Nutrition.* 2000;130 (6):1578-1583.

Brown L, Rimm EB, Seddon JM, et al. A prospective study of carotenoid intake and risk of cataract extraction in US men. *American Journal of Clinical Nutrition.* 1999;70(4):517-524.

Dewanto V, Wu X, Adom KK, Liu RH. Thermal processing enhances the nutritional value of tomatoes by increasing total antioxidant activity. *Journal of Agricultural Food Chemistry,* 2002; 8;50(10): 3010-4.

Elfhag K, Rossner S. Who succeeds in maintaining weight loss? A conceptual review of factors associated with weight loss maintenance and weight regain. *Obesity Reviews.* 2005;6(1):67-85.

Executive Summary: Conference on Dietary Supplement Use in the Elderly — Proceedings of the Conference Held January 14-15, 2003, Natcher Auditorium, National Institutes of Health, Bethesda, MD, Nutrition Reviews. 2004;62(4):160-175.

Farshchi HR, Taylor MA, Macdonald IA. Beneficial metabolic effects of regular meal frequency on dietary thermogenesis, insulin sensitivity, and

fasting lipid profiles in healthy obese women. *American Journal of Clinical Nutrition* 2005;81 (1):16-24.

Folsom, AR et al. Prospective study of coronary heart disease incidence in relation to fasting total homocysteine, related genetic polymorfism, and B vitamins. The atherosclerosis Risk in Communities (ARIC) study. *Circulation.* 1998; 98(3): 204-210.

Franzblau A, Rock CL, Werner RA, et al. The relationship of vitamin B6 status to median nerve function and carpal tunnel syndrome among active industrial workers. *Journal of Occupational and Environmental Medicine.* 1996;38(5):485-491.

Gianetti J, Pedrinelli R, Petrucci R, Lazzerini G, et al. Inverse association between carotid intimamedia thickness and the antioxidant lycopene in atherosclerosis. *American Heart Journal.* 2002;143 (3):467-474.

Godar D. UV Doses Worldwide. *Photochemistry and Photobiology.* 2005;81(4):736-749.

Gorin AA, Phelan S, Wing RR, Hill JO. Promoting long-term weight control: does dieting consistency matter? *International Journal Of Obesity and Related Metabolic Disorders.* 2004;28 (2):278-281.

Hanzlik RP, Fowler SC, Fisher DH. Relative bioavailability of calcium from calcium formate, calcium citrate and calcium carbonate. *Journal of Pharmacology and Experimental Therapeutics.* 2005; 313(3):1217-1222.

Harris JC, Cottrell SL, Plummer S, et al. Antimicrobial properties of Allium sativum (garlic). *Applied Microbiology and Biotechnology.* 2001;57(3):282-

286.

Heaney, RP, Rafferty K, Bierman J. Not all calcium fortified beverages are equal. *Nutrition Today*. 2005; 40(1):39-44.

Heber D, Bowerman S. *What Color is Your Diet?* New York, NY: Harper Collins/Regan, 2001.

Hemila H. Vitamin C supplementation and respiratory infections: a systematic review. *Military Medicine*. 2004;169 (11):920-925.

Hemila H. Vitamin C, respiratory infections and the immune system. *Trends in Immunology*. 2003;24(11):579-580.

Hodge AM, English DR, McCredie MR, et al. Foods, nutrients and prostate cancer. *Cancer Causes & Control*. 2004; 15(1):11-20.

Holick MF, Jenkins M. *The UV Advantage*. New York, NY: ibooks, inc, 2004.

Holick MF. Vitamin D: Importance in the prevention of cancers, type 1 diabetes, heart disease, and osteoporosis. *American Journal of Clinical Nutrition*. 2004; 79(3):362-371.

Holick MF. Sunlight and vitamin D for bone health and prevention of autoimmune diseases, cancers, and cardiovascular disease. *American Journal of Clinical Nutrition*. 2004;80(6 Suppl): 1678S-1688S.

Karanja NM, Obarzanek E, Lin PH, et al. Descriptive characteristics of the dietary patterns used in the Dietary Approaches to Stop Hypertension Trial. DASH Collaborative Research Group. *Journal of the American Dietetic Association*. 1999; 99: S19-S27.

Klem, ML, Wing, RR, McGuire, MT, et al. A descriptive study of individuals successful at long-term maintenance of substantial weight loss. *American Journal of Clinical Nutrition,* 1997, 66, 239-246.

Lila MA. Anthocyanins and Human Health: An In Vitro Investigative Approach. *Journal of Biomedicine & Biotechnology*. 2004;2004(5):306-313.

Mayo Foundation for Medical Education and Research, http://www.mayoclinic. com, accessed October 2005.

Mezzano D, Kosiel K, Martinez C, et al. Cardiovascular risk factors in vegetarians: normalization of hyperhomocysteinemia with vitamin B12 and reduction of platelet aggregation with n-3 fatty acids. *Thrombosis Research*. 2000;10093):153-160.

National Institutes of Health, Office of Dietary Supplements, http://ods.od.nih. gov/factsheets/vitamind.asp, accessed December 2005.

National Heart, Lung and Blood Institute, http://www.nhlbi.nih.gov/health/prof/heart/other/hm_sp01/nhbpep.htm, accessed October 2005.

Quiles JL, Ochoa JJ, Huertas JR, Mataix J. Coenzyme Q supplementation protects from age-related DNA double-strand breaks and increases lifespan in rats fed on a PUFA-rich diet. *Experimental gerontology*. 2004; 39(2):189-194.

Riso P, Visioli F, Erba D, et al. Lycopene and vitamin C concentrations increase in plasma and lymphocytes after tomato intake. Effects on cellular antioxidant protection. *European Journal of Clinical Nutrition*. 2004;58(10):1350-1358.

Ryan-Harshman M, Aldoori W Bone health. New role for vitamin K? *Canadian Family Physician.* 2004;50:993-997.

Ryan-Harshman M, Aldoori W. The relevance of selenium to immunity, cancer, and infectious/ inflammatory diseases. *Canadian Journal of Dietetic Practice and Research.* 2005;66(2):98-102.

Scagliusi, FB, Polacow VO, Artioli GG, et al. Selective underreporting of energy intake in women: magnitude, determinants, and effect of training. *Journal of the American Dietetic Association.* 2003;103(10):1306-13.

Tanyel MC, Mancano LD. Neurologic findings in vitamin E deficiency. *American Family Physician.* 1997;55(1):197-201.

Traber MG, Sies H. Vitamin E in humans: demand and delivery. *Annual Review of Nutrition.* 1996;16:321-347.

Zemel MB, Richards J, Mathis S, et al. Dairy augmentation of total and central fat loss in obese subjects. *International Journal Obesity.* 2005;29(4):391-397.

Zemel, MB, Miller SL. Dietary calcium and dairy modulation of adiposity and obesity risk. *Nutrition Reviews.* 2004; 62(4):125-31.

Activity Maps

Adams MA, Dolan P, Hutton WC. Diurnal variations in the stress on the lumbar spine. *Spine.* 1987;12(2):130-137.

Adlard PA, Cotman CW. Voluntary exercise protects against stress-induced decreases in brain-derived neurotrophic factor protein expression. *Neuro-science.* 2004;124(4):985-992.

Akerstedt T, Nilsson PM. Sleep as restitution: an introduction. *Journal of Internal Medicine.* 2003; 254(1):6-12.

Bailey RL, Ledikwe JH, Smiciklas-Wright H, et al. Persistent oral health problems associated with comorbidity and impaired diet quality in older adults. *Journal of the American Dietetic Association.* 2004;104(8):1273-1276.

Beasley R, Raymond N, Hill S, et al. eThrombosis: 21st Century variant of venous thromboembolism associated with immobility. *European Respiratory Journal.* 2003;21(2):374-376.

Berk LS, Felten DL, Tan SA, et al. Modulation of neuroimmune parameters during the eustress of humor-associated mirthful laughter. *Alternative Therapies In Health And Medicine.* 2001;7 (2):62-72, 74-76.

Bennett MP, Zeller JM, Rosenberg L, et al. The effect of mirthful laughter on stress and natural killer cell activity. *Alternative Therapies in Health and Medicine.* 2003;9(2):38-45.

Bode C, Bode JC. Effect of alcohol consumption on the gut. *Best Practice & Research. Clinical Gastroenterology.* 2003;17(4):575-592.

Borg G. *Borg's Perceived Exertion and Pain Scales.* Champaign, IL: Human Kinetics, 1998.

Calle EE, Rodriguez C, Walker-Thurmond K, et al. Overweight, obesity, and mortality from cancer in a prospectively studied cohort of U.S. adults. *New England Journal of Medicine.* 2003;348 (17):1625-1638.

Cassidy A. Diet and menopausal health. *Nursing*

Standard. 2005;19(29):44-52.

Clark WW. Noise exposure from leisure activities: A review. *Journal of the Acoustical Society of America*. 1991;90(1):175-181.

Clemente CD, ed. *Gray's Anatomy,* 13th ed. Philadelphia, PA: Lea & Febiger, 1985.

Coker KH. Meditation and prostate cancer: integrating a mind/body intervention with traditional therapies. *Seminars in Urologic Oncology.* 1999;17 (2):111-118.

Diabetes Prevention Program Research Group. Reduction in the Incidence of Type 2 Diabetes with Lifestyle Intervention or Metformin. *New England Journal of Medicine.* 2002;346(6):393-403.

Diabetes Prevention Program Research Group. The Diabetes Prevention Program: Design and methods for a clinical trial in the prevention of type 2 diabetes. *Diabetes Care.* 1999; 22(4):623-634.

Dixon JB, Schachter LM, O'Brien PE. Sleep disturbance and obesity: Changes following surgically induced weight loss. *Archives of Internal Medicine.* 2001;161(1):102-106.

Douglas S. Premenstrual syndrome. Evidence-based treatment in family practice. *Canadian Family Physician.* 2002;48:1789-1797.

Draelos ZD. The biology of hair care. *Dermatologic Clinics.* 2000; 18(4):651-658.

Evans JR, Fletcher AE, Wormald RP. 28 000 Cases of age related macular degeneration causing visual loss in people aged 75 years and above in the United Kingdom may be attributable to smoking. *British Journal of Ophthalmology.* 2005;89(5):550-553.

Forslund AH, El-Khoury AE, Olsson RM, et al. Effect of protein intake and physical activity on 24-h pattern and rate of macronutrient utilization. *American Journal of Physiology-Endocrinology and Metabolism.* 1999;276(5):E964-976.

Fortes C, Farchi S, Forastiere F, et al. Depressive symptoms lead to impaired cellular immune response. *Psychotherapy and Psychosomatics.* 2003;72(5):253-260.

Fujino T, Katou J, Fujita M, et al. Relationship between serum lipoprotein(a) level and thrombin generation to the circadian variation in onset of acute myocardial infarction. *Atherosclerosis.* 2001;155(1): 171-178.

Gavin J. Pairing personality with activity: New tools for inspiring active lifestyles. *Physician and Sportsmedicine.* 2004;32(12):17-24.

Giangrande PL. Air travel and thrombosis. *International Journal of Clinical Practice.* 2001;55 (10):690-693.

Giannopoulou I, Ploutz-Snyder LL, Carhart R, et al. Exercise is required for visceral fat loss in postmenopausal women with type 2 diabetes. *Journal Of Clinical Endocrinology And Metabolism.* 2005;90(3):1511-1518.

Girman A, Lee R, Kligler B. An integrative medicine approach to premenstrual syndrome. *American Journal of Obstetrics and Gynecology.* 2003;188(5 Suppl): S56-65.

Guccione AA. Arthritis. In: *Physical Rehabilitation: Assessment and Treatment,* 4th ed. O'Sullivan SB (ed), Schmitz TJ. Philadelphia, PA: F.A. Davis Company, 2001.

Hatano Y. Use of a pedometer for promoting daily walking exercise. *International Council for Health, Physical Education and Recreation.* 1993;26:649-660.

Haykowsky MJ, Eves ND, Warburton DE, et al. Resistance exercise, the valsalva maneuver, and cerebrovascular transmural pressure. *Medicine and Exercise in Sport and Exercise.* 2003;35 (1):65-68.

Heber D. *The Resolution Diet: Keeping the Promise of Permanent Weight Loss.* Garden City Park, NY: Avery Publishing Group, 1999.

Howley ET. You asked for it: Question authority (exercises in the morning after an overnight fast). *ACSM's Health & Fitness Journal.* 2001;5(6):5.

Katch FI, Clarkson PM, Kroll W, et al. Effects of sit-up exercise training on adipose cell size and adiposity. *Research Quarterly for Exercise and Sport.* 1984;55 (3):242-247.

Kollef MH, Neelon-Kollef RA. Pulmonary embolism associated with the act of defecation. *Heart and Lung.* 1991;20:451-454.

Krall EA, Wehler C, Garcia RI, et al. Calcium and vitamin D supplements reduce tooth loss in the elderly. *American Journal Of Medicine.* 2001;15; 111(6):452-456.

Kubesch S, Bretschneider V, Freudenmann R, et al. Aerobic endurance exercise improves executive functions in depressed patients. *The Journal of Clinical Psychiatry.* 2003;64 (9):1005-1012.

Laaksonen DE, Lindstrom J, Lakka TA, et al. Physical activity in the prevention of type 2 diabetes: the Finnish diabetes prevention study. *Diabetes.* 2005;54(1):158-165.

Leboeuf-Yde C. Body weight and low back pain. A systematic literature review of 56 journal articles reporting on 65 epidemiologic studies. *Spine.* 2000;25(2):226-237.

Leboeuf-Yde C, Kyvik KO, Bruun NH. Low back back pain and lifestyle. Part II: Obesity. Information from a population-based sample of 29,424 twin subjects. *Spine.* 1999;24(8):779-783.

Le Masurier GC, Sidman CL, Corbin CB. Accumulating 10,000 steps: Does this meet current physical activity guidelines? *Research Quarterly for Exercise and Sport.* 2003;74(4): 389-394.

Lembo A, Camilleri M. Chronic constipation. *New England Journal of Medicine.* 2003;349 (14):1360-1368.

Levine JA, Lanningham-Foster LM, McCrady SK, et al. Interindividual variation in posture allocation: Possible role in human obesity. *Science.* 2005;307(5709):584-586.

Levine JA, Eberhardt NL, Jensen MD. Role of nonexercise activity thermogenesis in resistance to fat gain in humans. *Science.* 1999;283(5399): 212-214.

Lytle ME, Vander Bilt J, Pandav RS, et al. Exercise level and cognitive decline: The MoVIES project. *Alzheimer Disease and Associated Disorders.* 2004;18 (2):57-64.

Major GC, Piche ME, Bergeron J, et al. Energy expenditure from physical activity and the metabolic risk profile at menopause. *Medicine & Science In Sports & Exercise.* 2005;37 (2):204-212.

Marcos A, Nova E, Montero A. Changes in the immune system are conditioned by nutrition.

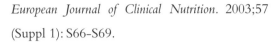

European Journal of Clinical Nutrition. 2003;57 (Suppl 1): S66-S69.

Marcus BH, Albrecht AE, King TK et al. The efficacy of exercise as an aid for smoking cessation in women: a randomized controlled trial. *Archives of Internal Medicine.* 1999;159(11):1229-1234.

Mclean L, Tingley M, Scott RN, et al. Computer terminal work and the benefit of microbreaks. *Applied Ergonomics.* 2001;32 (3):225-237.

Muller-Lissner SA, Kamm MA, Scarpignato C, et al. Myths and misconceptions about chronic constipation. *American Journal of Gastroenterology.* 2005;100(1): 232-242.

Nagata C, Hirokawa K, Shimizu N, et al. Soy, fat and other dietary factors in relation to premenstrual symptoms in Japanese women. *British Journal of Obstetrics and Gynaecology.* 2004;111(6):594-599.

Nieman DC. Current perspective on exercise immunology. *Current Sports Medicine Reports.* 2003;2(5):239-242.

O'Connell E. . Mood, energy, cognition, and physical complaints: a mind/body approach to symptom management during the climacteric. *Journal ff Obstetric, Gynecologic, And Neonatal Nursing.* 2005;34(2):274-279.

Osei-Tutu KB, Campagna PD. The effects of short- vs. long-bout exercise on mood, VO2max, and percent body fat. *Preventive Medicine.* 2005:40(1):92-98.

Oyabu T, Takenaka K, Wolverton B, et al. Purification characteristics of golden pothos for atmospheric gasoline. *International Journal of Phytoremediation.* 2003;5(3):267-276.

Peeke P, Chrousos GP. Hypercortisolism and obesity. *Annals of the New York Academy of Sciences.* 1995;771:665-676.

Peters HP, De Vries WR, Vanberge-Henegouwen GP, et al. Potential benefits and hazards of physical activity and exercise on the gastrointestinal tract. *Gut.* 2001;48(3):435-439.

Pierard GE, Nizet JL, Pierard-Franchimont C. Cellulite: From standing fat herniation to hypodermal stretch marks. *American Journal of Dermatopathology.* 2000;22 (1):34-37.

Pilates JH, Miller WJ. *Return to Life Through Contrology.* New York, NY: J.J. Augustin, 1945.

Pruett SB. Stress and the immune system. *Pathophysiology.* 2003;9 (3):133-153.

Purba MB, Kouris-Blazos A, Wattanapenpaiboon N, et al. Skin wrinkling: Can food make a difference? *Journal of the American College of Nutrition.* 2001;20 (1):71-80.

Reynolds LR, Anderson JW. Practical office strategies for weight management of the obese diabetic individual. 2004;10(2): 153-159.

Rushton DH. Nutritional factors and hair loss. *Clinical and Experimental Dermatology.* 2002;27 (5): 396-404.

Schaub B, von Mutius E. Obesity and asthma, what are the links? *Current Opinion in Allergy and Clinical Immunology.* 2005;5(2): 185-193.

Scherwitz C, Braun-Falco O. So-called cellulite. *Journal of Dermatologic Surgery and Oncology.* 1978;4:230-234.

Sheon RP, Orr PM. Appendix B: Joint protection guide for rheumatic disorders. In: *Soft Tissue*

Rheumatic Pain: Recognition, Management and Prevention, 3rd ed. Sheon RP, Moskowitz RW, Goldberg VM. Baltimore, MD: Williams & Wilkins, 1996.

Sikirov D. Comparison of straining during defecation in three positions. *Digestive Diseases and Sciences.* 2003;48(7):1201-1205.

Sizer F, Whitney E. *Nutrition: Concepts and Controversies,* 8th ed. Belmont, CA: Wadsworth/ Thomson Learning, 2000.

Small G. *The Memory Prescription: Dr. Gary Small's 14-Day Plan to Keep Your Brain and Body Young.* New York, NY: Hyperion, 2004.

Takahashi K, Iwase M, Yamashita K, et al. The elevation of natural killer cell activity induced by laughter in a crossover designed study. *International Journal of Molecular Medicine.* 2001;8(6):645-650.

Tanaka H, Shirakawa S. Sleep health, lifestyle and mental health in the Japanese elderly: Ensuring sleep to promote a healthy brain and mind. *Journal of Psychosomatic Research.* 2004; 56(5):465-477.

Tanne D, Medalie JH, Goldbourt U. Body fat distribution and long-term risk of stroke mortality. *Stroke.* 2005;36(5): 1021-1025.

Tepper S, McKeough D. Deep vein thrombosis: Risks, diagnosis, treatment intervention and prevention. *Acute Care Perspectives.* 2000;9(1):3-7.

Toda Y, Segal N, Toda T, et al. Lean body mass and body fat distribution in participants with chronic low back pain. *Archives of Internal Medicine.* 2000;160 (21):3265-3269.

Tudor-Locke C, Bassett DR Jr. How many steps/day are enough? Preliminary pedometer indices for public health. *Sports Medicine.* 2004;34(1):1-8.

Wang Y, Rimm EB, Stampfer MJ, et al. Comparison of abdominal adiposity and overall obesity in predicting risk of type 2 diabetes among men. *American Journal of Clinical Nutrition.* 2005;81 (3):555-563.

Zhu S, Heymsfield SB, Toyoshima H, et al. Race-ethnicity—specific waist circumference cutoffs for identifying cardio- vascular disease risk factors. *American Journal of Clinical Nutrition.* 2005; 81 (2):409-415.

Nutrition Diaries

The National Agricultural Library, www.nal.usda.gov, accessed November 2004

The Center for Science in the Public Interest, www.cspinet .org, accessed December 2004

The American Cancer Society, http://www.cancer.org/docroot/PED/content/PED_3_2X_Hints_for_Eating_Smart_with_Fruits_and_Vegetables.asp, accessed January 2005.

The American Heart Association, http://www.americanheart.org/presenter.jhtml, accessed February 2005.

The National Institutes of Health, http://ods.od.nih.gov/factsheets/calcium.asp, accessed March 2005.

The U.S. Department of Health and Human Services, http:// www.health.gov/dietaryguidelines, accessed March 2005.

Borek C. Dietary antioxidants and human cancer.

Integrative Cancer Therapies. 2004;3(4):333-341.

Cao G, Alessio HM, Cutler RG. Oxygen-radical absorbance capacity assay for antioxidants. *Free Radical Biology & Medicine.* 1993;14(3):303-11.

Cao G, Booth SL, Sadowski JA, et al. Increases in human plasma antioxidant capacity after consumption of controlled diets high in fruit and vegetables. *American Journal of Clinical Nutrition.* 1998 Nov;68(5): 1081-1087.

Dangour AD, Sibson VL, Fletcher AE. Micronutrient supplementation in later life: limited evidence for benefit. *Journals of Gerontology. Series A, Biological Sciences and Medical Sciences.* 2004;59(7):659-73.

Davis, RB, Turner LW. A review of current weight management: research and recommendations. *Journal of the American Academy of Nurse Practitioners.* 2001; 13(1): 15-19.

Demeule M, Michaud-Levesque J. Green tea catechins as novel antitumor and antiangiogenic compounds. *Current Medicinal Chemistry. Anti-Cancer Agents.* 2002;2(4):441-63.

Garcia-Lorda P, Megias Rangil I, Salas-Salvado J. Nut consumption, body weight and insulin resistance. *European Journal Of Clinical Nutrition.* 2003;57 (Suppl 1):S8-11.

Hodge AM, English DR, McCredie MR, et al. Foods, nutrients and prostate cancer. *Cancer Causes & Control.* 2004;15(1):11-20.

Jepson RG, Mihaljevic L, Craig J. Cranberries for preventing urinary tract infections. *Cochrane Database of Systematic Reviews.* 2004(2): CD001321.

Khan A, Safdar M, Khan MMA, et al. Cinnamon improves glucose and lipids of people with type 2 diabetes. *Diabetes Care.* 2003;26(12):3215-3218.

Lawrence ME, Kirby DF. Nutrition and sports supplements: Fact or fiction. *Journal of Clinical Gastroenterology.* 2002;35 (4): 299-306.

Lim GP, Chu T, Yang F, et al. The curry spice curcumin reduces oxidative damage and amyloid pathology in an Alzheimer transgenic mouse. *Journal of Neuroscience.* 2001;21(21):8370-8307.

Murray RK, Granner DK, Mayes PA, et al. *Harper's Biochemistry.* 25th Edition. Stamford, CT: Appleton and Lange, 2000.

Nicola PJ, Maradit-Kremers H et al. The risk of congestive heart failure in rheumatoid arthritis: a population-based study over 46 years. *Arthritis and Rheumatism.* 2005;52(2):412-420.

Shelmet JJ, Reichard GA, Skutches CL, et al. Ethanol causes acute inhibition of carbohydrate, fat, and protein oxidation and insulin resistance. *Journal of Clinical Investigation.* 1988;81 (4):1137-1145.

Shils ME, Olson JA, Shike M, et al. *Modern Nutrition in Health and Disease.* 9th Edition. Baltimore, MD: Williams and Wilkins, 1999.

Sonko BJ, Prentice AM, Murgatroyd PR, et al. Effect of alcohol on postmeal fat storage. *American Journal of Clinical Nutrition.* 1994;59(3):619-625.

Surh YJ, Park KK, Chun KS, et al. Anti-tumor-promoting activities of selected pungent phenolic substances present in ginger. *Journal of Environmental Pathology, Toxicology and Oncology.* 1999;18(2):131-139.

About the Authors

Z. Altug is a licensed physical therapist and fitness consultant. He works at the UCLA Medical Center as a physical therapist in the outpatient Rehabilitation Services Department and also designs fitness programs for busy professionals as a private fitness consultant. Z holds bachelor of science degrees in physical therapy and physical education and also a master of science degree in exercise science. A member of the American College of Sports Medicine, the National Strength and Conditioning Association, and the American Physical Therapy Association, he lives in Los Angeles, California and enjoys playing a variety of sports and traveling. Reach him at www.zaltug.com.

Tracy Olgeaty Gensler is a licensed registered dietitian. She is a health writer for consumer magazines and books and she speaks on a variety of nutrition topics. Tracy holds a bachelor of science degree in clinical nutrition and a master of science degree in nutrition education. She lives in Chevy Chase, Maryland with her husband and two daughters. Reach her at www.wellnesstowork.com.

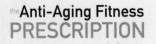
the **Anti-Aging Fitness**
PRESCRIPTION